Medical Library
Mercer University
School of Medicine
Macon, Ga 31207

Otto Krayer

# Rudolf Boehm
## and his School of Pharmacologists

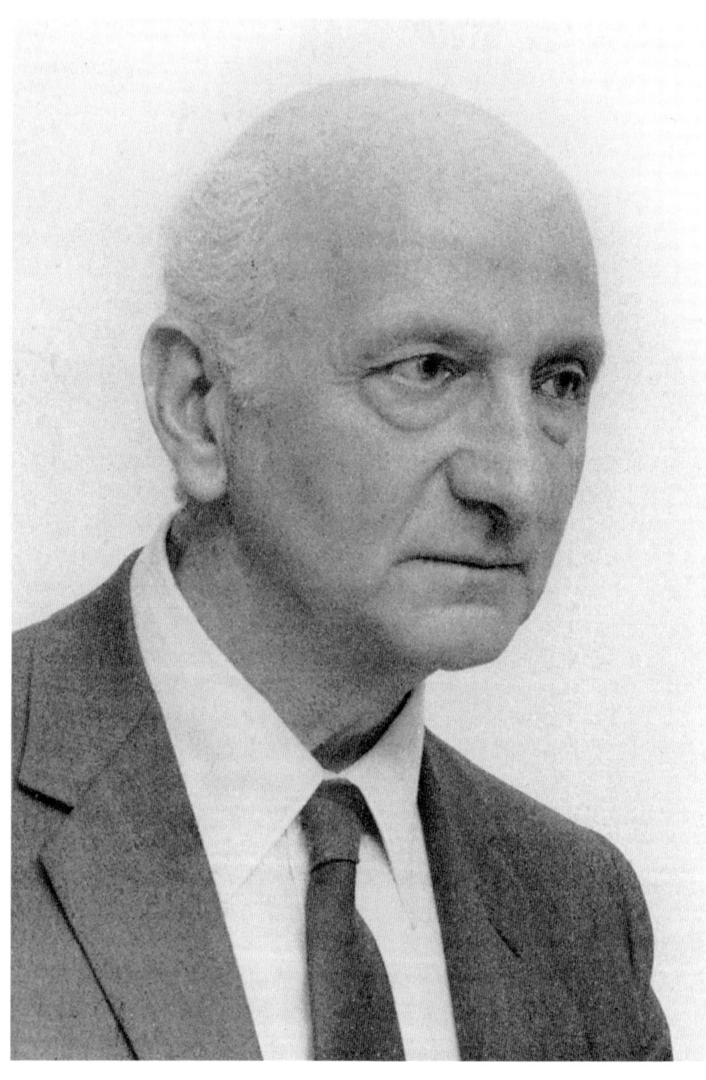


Otto Krayer.

# *Otto Krayer*

# Rudolf Boehm and his School of Pharmacologists

Edited by
Melchior Reiter

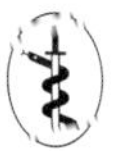

W. Zuckschwerdt Verlag München Bern Wien New York

German edition 1998, ISBN 3-88603-635-9

---

Distributors:

Germany:
Brockhaus Kommission
Verlagsauslieferung
Kreidlerstrasse 9
D-70806 Kornwestheim

Switzerland:
Hans Huber Verlag
Längassstrasse 76
CH-3000 Bern

Austria:
Maudrich Verlag
Spitalgasse 21a
A-1097 Wien

USA:
Scholium International Inc.
14 Vanderventer Ave
Port Washington
11050 NewYork

Die Deutsche Bibliothek – CIP-Einheitsaufnahme

**Krayer, Otto:** Rudolf Boehm and his school of pharmacologists / Otto Krayer. Ed. by Melchior Reiter.
- München ; Bern ; Wien ; New York : Zuckschwerdt, 1998
ISBN 3-88603-630-8

Trade-mark protection will not always be marked. The absence of a reference does not indicate an unprotected trade-mark.

All rights reserved. No part of this publication may be produced, stored in a retrieval system, or transmitted in any form or by any means, electronic, mechanical, photocopying, recording or otherwise, without prior permission from the publisher.

© 1998 by W. Zuckschwerdt Verlag GmbH, Industriestrasse 17, D-82110 Germering / München.
Printed in Germany by Presse-Druck Augsburg.

ISBN 3-88603-630-8

# Preface

Rudolf Buchheim was the founder of experimental pharmacology. In 1846, at the age of 26 he was appointed Professor of Materia Medica, Dietetics and History of Medicine in Dorpat. There he installed in his own house and from private means a laboratory for pharmacological investigation, which later became an institute of the univerity. Thus, Buchheim was the founder of the first department of pharmacology which, for two decades, remained the only one of its kind [1,2].

Buchheim's successor in Dorpat was his pupil Oswald Schmiedeberg who, soon after his appointment, took leave of absence for one year in 1871 in order to acquire "mastery in physiological

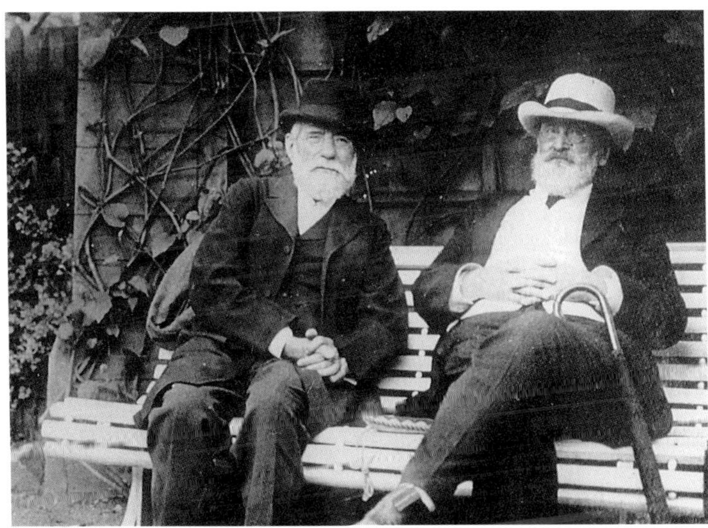

*Oswald Schmiedeberg and Rudolf Boehm*

experimentation" in the Department of Physiology at Leipzig under the directorship of Carl Ludwig[3]. Rudolf Boehm had also joined Carl Ludwig at that time with the same aim. The resulting friendship was probably not without influence on Boehm's nomination as head of the Dorpat department in 1872 after Schmiedeberg had been invited to the newly founded German University in Strassburg "on the warm recommendation of Carl Ludwig"[3].

Boehm moved to Marburg in 1881 and to Leipzig in 1884. Under his directorship the second centre of experimental pharmacological research in Germany, besides Strassburg[4], originated there.

We owe it to these two schools[5] that today pharmacology is not only an indispensable subject at medical school, but pharmacological institutions are also important places for biological research. This is true not only for the university departments but also for the pharmaceutical industry[6]. In the German-speaking areas about two thirds of the heads of pharmacology departments nominated in the first half of the 20th century belonged to one of the two schools[7], which are closely related with regard to the congruent concepts of their scientific aims and to their methodological roots.

Of Boehm's pupils, those who had directed their own departments for significant lengths of time were: Heffter, Straub, Gros, Schüller and Külz. To the second generation belong as pupils of Heffter: Bürgi and Keeser; of Straub: Führner, P. Trendelenburg, Forst and Weese; of Gros: Baur, Lendle, Hauschild and Hofmann; of Schüller: Hahn; and of Külz: Koll.

Otto Krayer, the author of this monograph, was a pupil of Paul Trendelenburg. Krayer left Germany in 1933 after a dispute with the Prussian Kultusministerium (Ministry of Education) concerning his refusal to take over the chair of pharmacology in Düsseldorf which had become vacant by the racially motivated dismissal of Professor Philipp Ellinger[8]. After a successful scientific career at the American University in Beirut [9] and at Harvard Medical School in Boston [10], Krayer moved to Tucson, Arizona, in 1971.

Krayer spent the summer months from 1972 to 1980 in München, as a visiting professor in the Department of Pharmacology and Toxicology of the Technical University, then directed by me. I first met Otto Krayer in 1948 on the occasion of his visiting München as the chairman of the Unitarian Service Committee Medical Mission to Germany [11]. With the help of the Rockefeller Foundation I worked in his department in Boston in 1949, from which lasting and close contacts ensued. During Krayer's stay in München another of his former coworkers, Ullrich Trendelenburg, the son of his teacher, taught at the neighbouring University of Würzburg. After Krayer's retirement he served as acting head of the Boston department, until he took over the chair in Würzburg.

Krayer used his stays in the München department to realize a plan he had entertained for a long time, namely to write a history of "Boehm's School", a project which dealt with the development of a substantial part of pharmacology in Germany from the second half of the 19th to the first half of the 20th century. The motive for his preoccupation with the history of his subject may be found in the wish to explore his scientific roots after thirty years at one of the leading universities of the "New World".

In accordance with his own genealogy, Krayer restricted himself to the presentation of Boehm and his pupils of the first generation as well as of Straub's pupils. Thus, only a small section of Boehm's school is represented here; but this presentation gains in scientific-historical importance through the eminence of Straub's personality and the achievements of his pupils.

By 1979 the manuscript had progressed to the point where Krayer was able to give seminars on Boehm and several of his pupils, in München as well as to the graduate students of the Department of Pharmacology directed by his pupil W. Flacke in Little Rock, Arkansas. He avoided discussions concerning the eventual publication of his manuscript. He still regarded his treatment of the topic as too superficial and incomplete, "basically not more than a study of my pharmacological forebears".

Early in 1982 Krayer died in Tuscon without having made any decision about the future of his manuscript. With the help of his widow, Dr. Erna Ruth Krayer, and Ullrich Trendelenburg, it was possible to transfer the material in Tucson and to unite it with the material in München.

As Krayer's local trustee I regarded it as an obligation to complete the project he began and to make it available to the public at large.

When the material was prepared for publication, certain gaps were filled in accordance with Krayer's intentions, such as in the chapters on Gros, Schüller, Fühner, Forst and Weese. With the exception of the chapter on Paul Trendelenburg, Krayer had written his manuscripts in German; most of the final versions were then translated into English in Tucson. The bilingual format has been retained. Missing translations were supplied by Ullrich Trendelenburg, kindly supported by Dr. John R. Fozard.

Finally, it appeared appropriate to add to "Boehm's School" an overview of the scientific work of Otto Krayer as well as his curriculum vitae, especially since authentic texts were available from Krayer's estate. These two manuscripts appear here unchanged.


*Melchior Reiter*


München, November 1997

1 SCHMIEDEBERG, O. (1912). Rudolf Buchheim, sein Leben und seine Bedeutung für die Begründung der wissenschaftlichen Arzneimittellehre und Pharmakologie. Arch. exp. Path. Pharmakol., 67, 1-54.

2 HABERMANN, E. R. (1974). Rudolf Buchheim and the Beginning of Pharmacology as a Science. Annual Rev. Pharmacol., 14, 1-8.

3 HEFFTER, A. (1922). II. Rede des antretenden Rektors A. Heffter: Buchheim und Schmiedeberg, die Begründer der experimentellen Pharmakologie. Rektorwechsel an der Friedrich-Wilhelm-Universität zu Berlin am 15. Oktober 1922. 9-14. Berlin: Norddeutsche Buchdruckerei und Verlagsanstalt A. G.

4 KOCH-WESER, J. & SCHECHTER, J. P. (1978). Schmiedeberg in Strassburg 1872-1918: The Making of Modern Pharmacology. Life Sciences, 22, 1361-1372.

5 MUSCHOLL, E. (1995). The evolution of experimental pharmacology as a biological science: the pioneering work of Buchheim and Schmiedeberg. Brit. J. Pharmacol., 116, 2155-2159.

6 THOMAS, K. (1926). Nachruf auf Rudolf Boehm, Ber. d. Math. Phys. Klasse d. sächs. Akad d. Wiss. zu Leipzig, LXXVIII, 348-357.

7 LINDNER, J. (1957). Zeittafeln zur Geschichte der pharmakologischen Institute des deutschen Sprachgebietes. 167 pp., Aulendorf i. Württ.: Editio Cantor.

8 TRENDELENBURG, U. (1995). Otto Krayer und das „Gesetz zur Wiederherstellung des Berufsbeamtentums" (April 1933). DGPT Mitteilungen Nr. 16, 33-34. Stuttgart: Wissenschaftliche Verlagsgesellschaft.

9 FAWAZ, G. (1983). Cornerstones. A rare bird of passage alights on the AUB campus and stays on for three years. Otto Krayer (1899-1982) as I knew him. Medicus, 15, 10-15

10 GOLDSTEIN, A. (1987). Otto Krayer 1899-1982. A Biographical Memoir. Biographical Memoirs, 57, 151-225. Washington, D. C.: The National Academy Press.

11 LECTURES - Unitarian Service Committee Medical Mission to Germany, July 2 - September 3, 1948, ed. O. Krayer (1950). 312 pp., Berlin: Springer.

X

---

# Contents

# XII

---

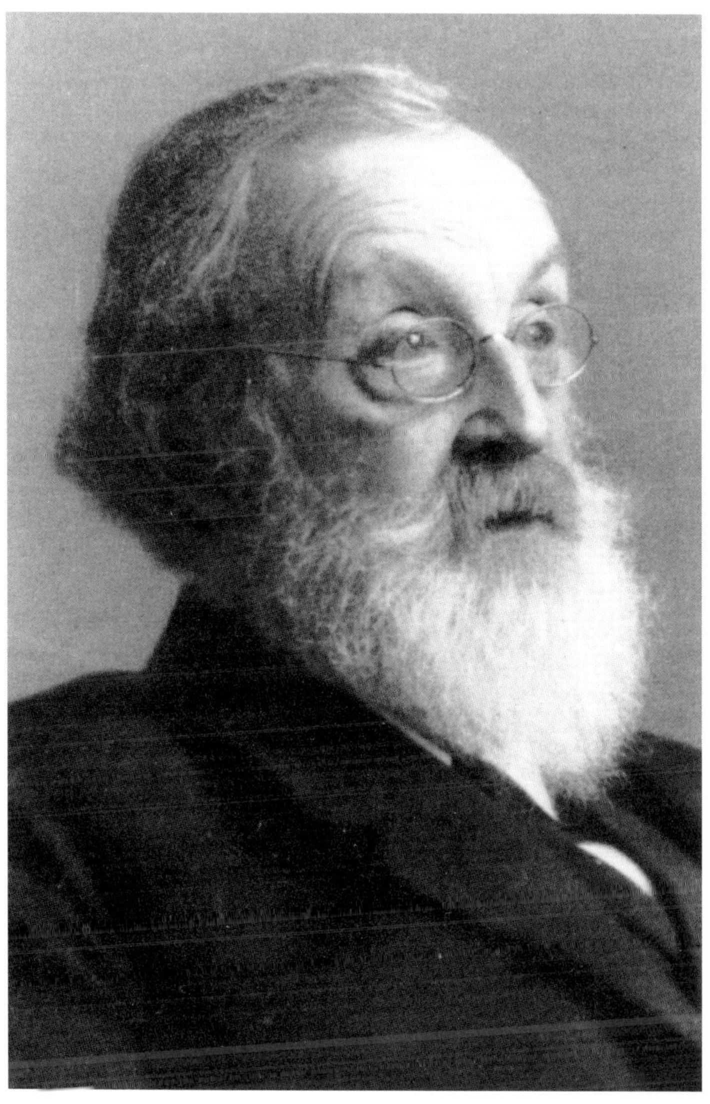

*Rudolf Boehm*

# Rudolf Boehm
## 1844 – 1926[*]



Rudolf Boehm was born on May 19, 1844 at Nördlingen in Bavaria, Germany. His father was district physician. Boehm studied medicine at the Universities of München, Würzburg and Leipzig where he received on Aug. 7, 1867 his medical degree (Dr. med.). While a medical student at Würzburg he participated in experimental studies in the Department of Pathology under von Recklinghausen. It was the desire of his father that Boehm should enter a clinical field that made him to start a two-year postdoctoral training in psychiatry as an Assistant to the Professor of Psychiatry of Würzburg University Franz von Rinecker. Von Rinecker was a scientist with broad interests who, besides psychiatry, had taught other branches of medical science including Materia Medica. He soon recognized the propensity of his assistant for experimental investigations. Moreover, he supported it and it was probably due to von Rinecker's suggestion that, in 1870, Boehm decided to strengthen the foundation of knowledge and deepen his physiological training by entering the physiological laboratory of Carl Ludwig at the University of Leipzig. There Boehm made the acquaintance of a remarkable group of outstanding young scientists, among them G. Hüfner, F. Miescher, O. Schmiedeberg. In this Leipzig period Boehm began to investigate on the frog heart in situ the effect of several alkaloids and alkaloid mixtures, i.e., atropine and muscarine, nicotine, aconitine, delphinine, veratrine, physostigmine and coniine. After a few months this work was interrupted by the outbreak of the Franco-Prussian war 1870–71 during which Boehm served as physician of a Bavarian battalion.

---

[*] Biographical sources: Heffter, 1914; Fühner, 1924; Thomas, 1926; Schüller, 1926; Gelbke, 1956; Lindner, 1957.

After the war Boehm returned to Würzburg University as an Assistant in the Department of Physiology under A. Fick. He completed the studies on cardiac poisons begun in Ludwig's laboratory and published the results (Boehm, 1871). In 1871 he also qualified for inauguration as academic Lecturer in Physiology. Partly in collaboration with Fick and partly together with pupils of his own, investigations were carried out on the action of veratrine upon skeletal muscle, on the action of aconitine, and on the influence of arsenic on fermentation. Of interest are experiments with digitalis preparations Boehm conducted at this time on the isolated heart of the frog. The heart was perfused from the venous side and the ventricle emptied through a cannula inserted into the bulb of the aorta against a variable resistance. Boehm had become familiar with this preparation while working in Ludwig's laboratories. He measured the work of the heart and its alteration by digitalis. These and other experiments led Boehm to the conclusion that the improvement of the work performance of the heart by small doses of digitalis represents the fundamental therapeutic effect (Boehm, 1872).

Already in 1872, Boehm took over the professorship of Pharmacology, Dietetics and History of Medicine at Dorpat in Estonia. There he succeeded his friend Oswald Schmiedeberg who, earlier in 1872, had been called to the chair of Pharmacology in the newly established University of Strassburg. From Dorpat there were several publications of his pupils, dealing with pharmacological topics. Boehm himself (1876a) clarified the biological effect of water hemlock (Cicuta virosa) He isolated the resinous active principle, cicutoxin, and found it to cause convulsions similar to those produced by picrotoxin. Together with the clinician F. A. Hoffmann, Boehm investigated problems dealing with the carbohydrate metabolism, i.e., the glycogen content and its utilization in the animal organism and the diabetes occurring in cats when the animals are restrained (Fesselungsdiabetes). By himself he examined the glycogen content of skeletal muscle in rigor mortis and showed that rigor mortis occurs without disappearance of glycogen. During the Dorpat period Boehm also made his first critical literary contribution to pharmacology and toxicology in the "Handbuch der Intoxikationen", edited by him jointly with B. Naunyn and H. v. Boeck, in which he treated the poisonous effects of the halogens, acids, alkalis, alkaline earths, the intoxication by anaesthetics and other aliphatic and mono-cyclic organic compounds, and the poisoning by spoiled food stuffs, especially botulism (Boehm, 1876b).

From 1881 to 1884 Boehm was Professor of Pharmacology at the University of Marburg. During this period his scientific interest centered on the poisonous principles of mushrooms. Together with one of his pupils he isolated from edible morel (Helvella esculenta) its poisonous substance, helvellic acid. Boehm himself examined a series of basidiomycytous mushrooms (Hutpilze, Boehm, 1885a) in which he found muscarine, as Schmiedeberg and Koppe (1869) had found it in fly agaric, Agaricus muscarius L. (Amanita muscaria). In subsequent studies on choline and on synthetic muscarins Boehm (1885b) discovered their "action upon nerve endings" (the peripheral postsynaptic action) which he examined more closely. As a result he concluded that the "synthetic muscarine" prepared according to Schmiedeberg and Harnack (1876) by the action of nitric acid on choline could not be identical with the natural muscarine. Contrary to the natural muscarine, the synthetic substance did not only have the characteristic "action on nerve endings" but, in higher doses, also exhibited a curare-like action upon skeletal muscle.

In 1884 Boehm was called to the chair of Pharmacology at the University of Leipzig. At first he and his pupils had to content themselves with small rooms and limited facilities. However, between 1886 and 1888 a new building was erected which contained laboratories and teaching facilities according to Boehm's own design and exemplary for that time. He directed his department until his retirement in 1921. He died in Bad Kohlgrub, Upper Bavaria, on August 19, 1926.

As an Assistant in Physiology at Leipzig University under Ludwig and at Würzburg University under Fick who, in 1868, had succeeded A. von Bezold, Boehm had become acquainted with biologically active plant extracts and mixtures of active principles of various medicinal plants, e.g., curare, veratrine, aconitine. At Dorpat and later at Marburg he chemically investigated different plants in the quest for the active principles. When Boehm took over the chair of Pharmacology at the University of Leipzig his interest in botany and his increasingly developing trend to work with chemical and physicochemical methods received a new and strong impulse. In contrast to most other German Universities, at Leipzig it belonged to the customary tasks of the Professor of Pharmacology not only to teach pharmacology to medical students but also to instruct the students of pharmacy in the field of pharmacognosy. Boehm dedicated the same devotion and care to both tasks. Very probably it was the intensive occupation with pharmacognosy and its for Boehm most important part pharmacochemistry which contributed in a large measure to the fact that Boehm became one of the leading pharmacologists of his time who, following the example of Sertürner, examined numerous plants and plant extracts for their chemically pure active constituents which are responsible for the pharmacological or toxicological activity. At Leipzig University from 1884 to his retirement in 1921, and beyond this to his death in 1926, Boehm directed and actively participated in a series of systematic investigations on the active constituents of medicinal substances containing vermifuges, cathartics, bitter and tanning substances, on alkaloid plants and on arrow poisons.

Boehm had great success in the very difficult investigation of the vermifuge drugs, especially of the extract of Filix mas. He discovered filix acid and various other crystalline substances, clarified their relation to each other and determined their chemical structure (Boehm, 1897). The active principles of Filix extract turned out to be complex homologues of phloroglucin. Several other vermifuges, e.g., Rhizoma Pannae, Flores Koso, Kamala, contained substances with similar structures, as Boehm and his coworkers found. So he had succeeded to show in a new example, what had been known already for the caffeine-containing drugs, that the natives in different parts of the world had by themselves found and utilized in different plant families those parts of the plant with the same pharmacological activity (literature, see Straub, 1924).

The investigations on alkaloid-bearing drugs concerned Folia Belladonnae, Radix Ipecacuanhae, Rhizoma Veratri, Semen Sabadillae, Nicotiana Tabacum and various cacti. Boehm's interest in the veratrum alkaloids led to the isolation of a new alkaloid, protoveratrine, from rhizome of veratrum album by his pupil Salzberger (1890). Protoveratrine (which we know is a mixture of two chemically closely related alkaloids, protoveratrine A and protoveratrine B), the alkaloid mixture veratrine from Semen Sabadillae, and cevadine, one of its pure constituent alkaloids, were studied pharmacolocically by Boehm and two of his pupils. Of the various species of cacti, which were examined chemically and pharmacologically especially by Boehm's pupil, Arthur Heffter, the active principles of the Peyote Cacti, e.g., mescaline, have remained of great interest (Heffter, 1898; Joachimoglu and Keeser, 1924).

Already at Dorpat, Boehm had realized that curare, which had become so important and valuable for physiological investigations, was of extremely varied composition. For over a decade he occupied himself with the subject. He clarified the origins of various kinds of curare, and he initiated the chemical investigation. Evidence for this can be found in his earliest publications in which he reported on the classification of the types (Sorten) of curare and on the isolation of different amorphous "curarines" (Boehm, 1895, 1898). Boehm's occupation over many years with curare and the curare alkaloids found a literary expression in his comprehensive review of the older literature in Heffter's Handbuch der experimentellen Pharmakologie (Boehm, 1920a). There he also published thorough reviews on the older literature concerning the chemistry and pharmacology of the veratrum alkaloids (Boehm, 1920b) and on the aconitum alkaloids (Boehm, 1920c).

In his lectures to students of medicine Boehm emphasized not only the experimental pharmacological research, but also therapeutics, the clinical experience with drugs. Boehm's lectures and demonstrations must have been very stimulating, as his American pupil J. J. Abel testified who, in 1884–86, had been in Leipzig where he took Boehm's course before he went to Strassburg to Schmiedeberg where he obtained his Dr.med. in 1888. That Boehm had interest in, and understanding for, the requirements of the practice of medicine found an expression also in his textbook on the Prescription of Drugs which appeared in three editions (Boehm, 1884).

# References

BOEHM, R. (1871). Studien über Herzgifte. 96 pp., 1 Tafel. Würzburg: A. Stubers Buchhandlung.

BOEHM, R. (1872). Untersuchungen über die physiologische Wirkung der Digitalis und des Digitalin. Pflügers Arch. ges. Physiol., 5, 153-191.

BOEHM, R. (1876a). Über den giftigen Bestandteil des Wasserschierlings (Cicuta virosa) und seine Wirkungen; ein Beitrag zur Kenntnis der Krampfgifte. Arch. exp. Path. Pharmakol., 5, 279-310.

BOEHM, R. (1876b). Handbuch der Intoxikationen, ed. by Boehm, R., Naunyn, B., and Boeck, H. v.. In H.v. Ziemssens Handb. d. Spez. Path. u. Therapie, 15, 1-252. Leipzig: F.C.W. Vogel.

BOEHM, R. (1884). Lehrbuch der allgemeinen und speziellen Arzneiverordnungslehre. 676 pp., 2. Auflage 1891. 491 pp., 3. Auflage 1903. 334 pp., Jena: Gustav Fischer.

BOEHM, R. (1885a). Beiträge zur Kenntnis der Hutpilze in chemischer und toxikologischer Beziehung. Arch. exp. Path. Pharmakol., 19, 60-86.

BOEHM, R. (1885b). Über das Vorkommen und die Wirkungen des Cholins und die Wirkungen der künstlichen Muscarine. Arch. exp. Path. Pharmakol., 19, 87-100.

BOEHM, R. (1897). Beitrag zur Kenntnis der Filixsäuregruppe. Arch. exp. Path. Pharmakol., 38, 35-58.

BOEHM, R. (1895, 1898). Das südamerikanische Pfeilgift Curare in chemischer und pharmakologischer Beziehung. I. Teil: Das Tubocurare. II. Teil: 1. Das Kalebassencurare, 2. Das Topfcurare, 3. Über einige Curarerinden. In Abhdl. d. Kgl. Sächs. Ges d. Wissenschaften, Math.-Phys. Classe, 22, 201-238, 1 Tafel; 24, 1-52, 4 Tafeln. Leipzig.

BOEHM, R. (1920a). Curare und Curarealkaloide.In Heffters Handb. exp. Pharmakol., 2, Teil I, 179-248. Berlin: Springer.

BOEHM, R. (1920b). Veratrin und Protoverartrin.In Heffters Handb. exp. Pharmakol., 2, Teil I, 249-282. Berlin: Springer.

BOEHM, R. (1920c). Die Aconitingruppe. In Heffters Handb. exp. Pharmakol., 2, Teil I, 283-319. Berlin: Springer.

FÜHNER, H. (1924). Rudolf Boehm und die Pharmakognosie. Pharmazeutische Ztg., 69, 471.

GELBKE, N. (1956). Die geschichtliche Entwicklung des Pharmakologischen Instituts der Leipziger Universität unter besonderer Berücksichtigung der Gründerjahre. Inaugural-Diss., Leipzig.

HEFFTER, A. (1898). Über Pellote. Beiträge zur chemischen und pharmakologischen Kenntnis der Cacteen. 2. Mitteilung. Arch. exp. Path. Pharmakol., 40, 385-429.

HEFFTER, A. (1914). Zu Rudolf Boehm's 70. Geburtstage. Berliner klin. Wschr., No. 20, 962-963.

JOACHIMOGLU, G. & KEESER, E. (1924). Kakteenalkaloide. In Heffters Handb. exp. Pharmakol., 2, Teil II, 1104-1113. Berlin: Springer.

LINDNER, J. (1957). Zeittafeln zur Geschichte der pharmakologischen Institute des deutschen Sprachgebietes. Aulendorf i. Württ.: Editio Cantor.

SALZBERGER, G. (1890). Über die Alkaloide der weißen Nieswurz (Veratrum album). Arch. Pharmazie, 228, 462-483.

SCHMIEDEBERG, O. & HARNACK, E. (1876). Über die Synthese des Muscarins und über muscarinartig wirkende Ammoniumbasen. Arch. exp. Path. Pharmakol., 6, 101-112.

SCHMIEDEBERG, O. & KOPPE, R. (1869). Das Muscarin, das giftige Alkaloid des Fliegenpilzes (Agaricus muscarius L.). 111 pp., Leipzig: F.C.W. Vogel.

SCHÜLLER, J. (1926). Rudolf Boehm. Münch. med. Wschr.,73/II, 2170.

STRAUB, W. (1924). Die Filixgruppe. In Heffters Handb. exp. Pharmakol. 2, Teil II, 1548-1562. Berlin: Springer.

THOMAS, K. (1926). Nachruf auf Rudolf Boehm. In Berichte Verhandl. Sächs. Akad. d. Wissenschaften zu Leipzig. Math.-Phys. Klasse. 78, 348-357.

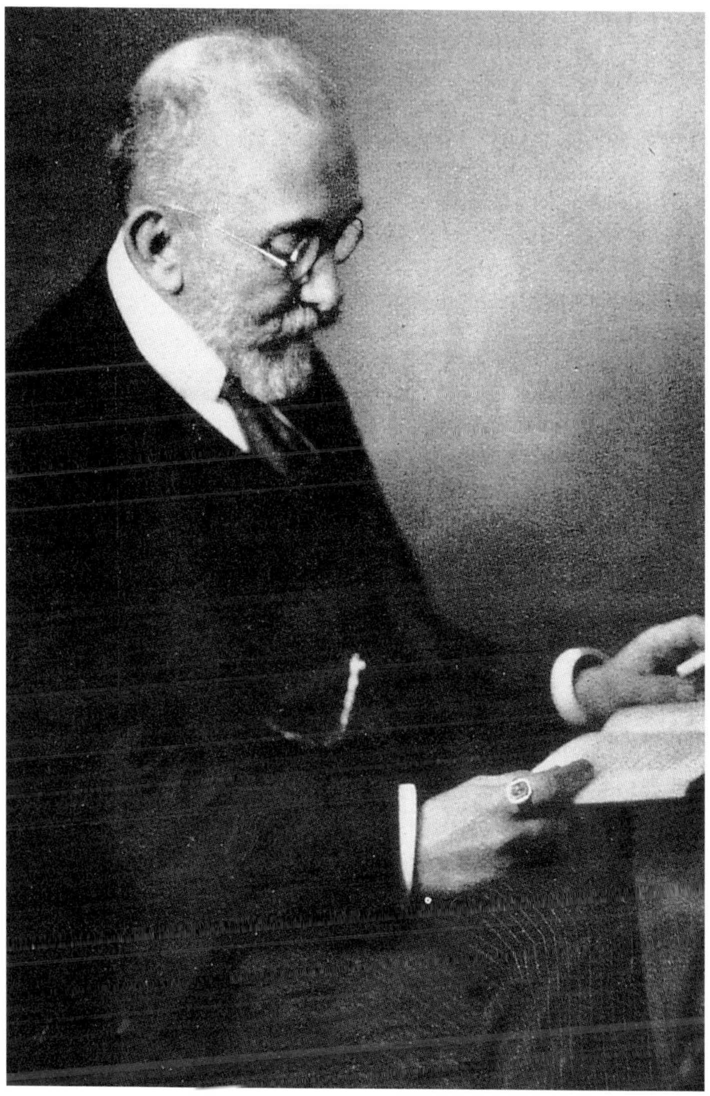

*Arthur Heffter*

# Arthur Heffter
# 1859 – 1925 [*]

Arthur Heffter was born in Leipzig on July 15, 1859 as the only child of a merchant family. After graduating from high school he studied chemistry at Freiburg, Leipzig and finally at Greifswald University, where, in 1883, he received the degree of Dr. phil. (Ph.D.). After a brief period as a chemist at the Agricultural-chemical Experimental Station at Halle he joined Otto F. J. Nasse at the University of Rostock where, in 1880, Nasse had become head of the Department of Pharmacology and Physiological Chemistry. During his assistantship, from 1884–1886, Heffter jointly with Nasse carried out his first scientific investigation 'on primary and secondary oxidations' (Nasse and Heffter, 1887). On his own Heffter investigated the excretion of sulfur in the urine and made the important observation that, in protein solutions, elementary sulfur is reduced to hydrogen sulfide (Heffter, 1886).

Heffter's interest in medicine caused him to enrol as a medical student at the University of Leipzig where, in 1896, he received his M.D. degree. While a student of medicine he was also engaged in research work at the laboratory of Pharmacology under Rudolf Boehm. A fruit of his endeavours was the synthesis, from chloral hydrate and glucose, of a new compound, chloralose. Heffter also investigated the pharmacological properties of chloralose which has remained an important general anaesthetic agent for animal experimentation. After his promotion Heffter spent a six month period at the pharmacological laboratory of Schmiedeberg at Strassburg University and then returned to

---

[*] Biographical sources: Straub, 1925; Heubner, 1925, 1927a; Lindner, 1957; Joachimoglu, 1960.

Leipzig University as an Assistant to Boehm. According to Straub (1925) joining Boehm's laboratory was of decisive importance for Heffter's development as a pharmacologist. In 1892 he qualified for inauguration as a Lecturer in Pharmacology and in 1896 he received the title of Professor. In 1898 Heffter was appointed Pharmacologist at the Department of Health of the German Government (Reichsgesundheitsamt) in Berlin but relinquished this position in the same year to accept the call to the chair of Medicinal Chemistry and Pharmacology at the University of Bern (Switzerland). In 1906 Heffter returned to Germany and, after a brief period as Professor of Pharmacology and head of the department at Marburg University, he was called to the University of Berlin in 1908. He remained director of its Department of Pharmacology until the time of his death in 1925.

Heffter's methods of work were essentially chemical. He was especially attracted by the field of pharmacochemistry. In Boehm's laboratory he isolated from Radix Pannae the active constituents related to filix acid (Heffter, 1897). There originated also his first publication on the alkaloids of cacti (Heffter, 1894, 1898) which were later continued (Joachimoglu and Keeser, 1924). Of special importance are Heffter's investigations of various species of anhalonium. From Anhalonium Lewinii he was able to isolate several alkaloids. Moreover, in experiments on himself he succeeded in identifying mescaline as the active principle which is responsible for the most important symptoms of poisoning with peyote and mescal, i.e., especially the unique colour visions and the loss of sense of time. These self experiments with pure substances he had isolated himself made Heffter one of the founders of scientific psychopharmacology in man. Heffter made also important contributions to the isolation of the strophanthins (Heffter and Sachs, 1912).

Heffter's attention was directed especially to the problems of uptake, distribution and elimination of drugs in the organism of animals and man. In regard to these aspects of general pharmacology, Heffter and his pupils investigated in great detail e. g. sulfur, arsenic, iodine and mercury. It is of interest in this connection that, when P. Ehrlich in developing his concepts on chemotherapy and chemoreceptors assumed that hydroxyl groups might be responsible for the selective binding, it was Heffter who drew his attention to the sulfhydryl groups which in all probability were the binding sites for his arsenic compounds and thereby opened the way to understanding of the selective therapeutic effect of this group of substances (Ehrlich, 1909).

During the 16 years of serving as Professor of Pharmacology at Berlin University Heffter devoted a great deal of his efforts to the task of an expert advisor for the Public Health System. Problems concerning industrial toxicology, food chemistry, intentional or malicious poisoning caused civil and military authorities to seek his advice. An excellent and important example of this kind of work and of the care with which it was carried out is his series of investigations into the evaluation of chemically identified amounts of arsenic found in corpses (Heffter, 1918). Walther Straub, a friend of Heffter's, had this to say: "When, today, the jurisdiction is cognizant of the fact that the presence of arsenic in hair and bone does not suffice to assume a dolus [Lat.]; when one can now state with assurance that the presence of arsenic in hair and bone of cadavers only proves a long-lasting medical administration of small and non-toxic doses of arsenic compounds and when just sentences can now be passed, it must be recognized that the credit for this is due to Heffter's quiet, critical scientific work".

In the literary domain Heffter made outstanding contributions to the growth of reliable pharmacological and toxicological knowledge by carefully prepared editorial reviews. In 'Schmidt's Jahrbücher der gesamten Medizin' there is a series of comprehensive critical reports on German and foreign toxicological publications covering a decade (Heffter, 1896, 1898, 1901, 1903; Heffter and Loeb, 1907). In 'Ergebnisse der Physiologie' he reported on the excretion in the urine of "körperfremder" substances foreign to the human organism (Heffter, 1902, 1903, 1905). Of even greater importance for scientific pharmacology is the work of Heffter as initiator and first editor of the Handbuch der experimentellen Pharmakologie (Handbook of experimental Pharmacology) which bears his name. In this handbook appeared posthumously Heffter's comprehensive reviews on his own areas of scientific work, i.e., "Arsen und seine Verbindungen" (Heffter and Keeser, 1927), "Phosphor und Phosphorverbindungen" (Heffter, 1927). The work of Heffter on the pharmacology of sulfur was extensively discussed in the handbook by W. Heubner in a review on sulfur (Heubner, 1927b). It was W. Heubner who succeeded Heffter as editor of the Handbuch der experimentellen Pharmakologie.

## References

EHRLICH, P. (1909). Über den jetzigen Stand der Chemotherapie. Ber. deutsch. Chem. Ges., 42, 17-47.

HEFFTER, A. (1886). Die Ausscheidung des Schwefels im Harn. Pflügers Arch. ges. Physiol., 38, 476-502.

HEFFTER, A. (1894). Über Pellote. Ein Beitrag zur pharmakologischen Kenntnis der Cacteen. Arch. exp. Path. Pharmakol., 34, 65-86.

HEFFTER, A. (1896-1907). Berichte über toxikologische Arbeiten aus den Jahren 1894-1906. Schmidts Jahrbücher der in- und ausländischen gesamten Medicin:
(1896). 249, 19-27; 125-138; 239-242.
(1898). 257, 91-101; 189-210.
(1901). 270, 9 25; 151-162.
(1903). 278, 14-27; 130-138.
(1907). 294, 1-9; 113 124. [HEFFTER & LOEB]

HEFFTER, A. (1897). Über einige Bestandteile von Rhizoma Pannae. Ein Beitrag zur Kenntnis der Filixsäuregruppe. Arch. exp. Path. Pharmakol., 38, 458-469.

HEFFTER, A. (1898). Über Pellote. Beiträge zur chemischen und pharmakologischen Kenntnis der Cacteen. 2. Mitteilung. Arch. exp. Path. Pharmakol., 40, 385-429.

HEFFTER, A. (1902). Chemie des Harns. Erg. Physiol., 1, 438-463.

HEFFTER, A. (1903). Ausscheidung körperfremder Substanzen im Harn. I. Teil. Erg. Physiol., 2, 95-129.

HEFFTER, A. (1905). Ausscheidung körperfremder Substanzen im Harn. II. Teil. Erg. Physiol., 4, 184-306.

HEFFTER, A. (1918). Giftmord oder Tod durch fortgesetzte freiwillige Arsenikzufuhr? Arch. f. Kriminologie., 70, 163-176.

HEFFTER, A. (1927). Phosphor und Phosphorverbindungen. In Heffters Handb. exp. Pharmakol., 3, Teil I, 568-619. Berlin: Springer.

HEFFTER, A. & KEESER, E. (1927). Arsen und seine Verbindungen. In Heffters Handb. exp. Pharmakol., 3, Teil I, 463-532. Berlin: Springer.

HEFFTER, A. & SACHS, F. (1912). Vergleichende Untersuchungen über Strophanthus-Glucoside. Biochem. Z., 40, 83-124.

HEUBNER, W. (1925). Nachruf auf Arthur Heffter. Zentralblatt Gew. Hyg. u. Unfallverhütung, N.F., 2, 101-103.

HEUBNER, W. (1927a). Vorwort zum dritten Band. In Heffters Handb. exp. Pharmakol., 3, Teil I, V-VII. Berlin: Springer.

HEUBNER, W. (1927b). Schwefel. In Heffters Handb. exp. Pharmakol., 3, Teil I, 418-432.

JOACHIMOGLU, G. (1960). Eröffnungsansprache (zum 100. Geburtstage von Arthur Heffter). Arch. exp. Path. Pharmakol., 238, 6-7.

JOACHIMOGLU, G. & KEESER, E. (1924). Kakteenalkaloide. In Heffters Handb. exp. Pharmakol., 2, Teil II, 1104-1113. Berlin: Springer.

LINDNER, J. (1957). Zeittafeln zur Geschichte der pharmakologischen Institute des deutschen Sprachgebietes. 167 pp., Aulendorf i. Württ.: Editio Cantor.

NASSE, O. & HEFFTER, A. (1887). Über primäre und sekundäre Oxydationen. Pflügers Arch. ges. Physiol., 41, 378-389.

STRAUB, W. (1925). Arthur Heffter, Nachruf. Arch. exp. Path. Pharmakol., 105, I-IV between pp. 264 and 265.

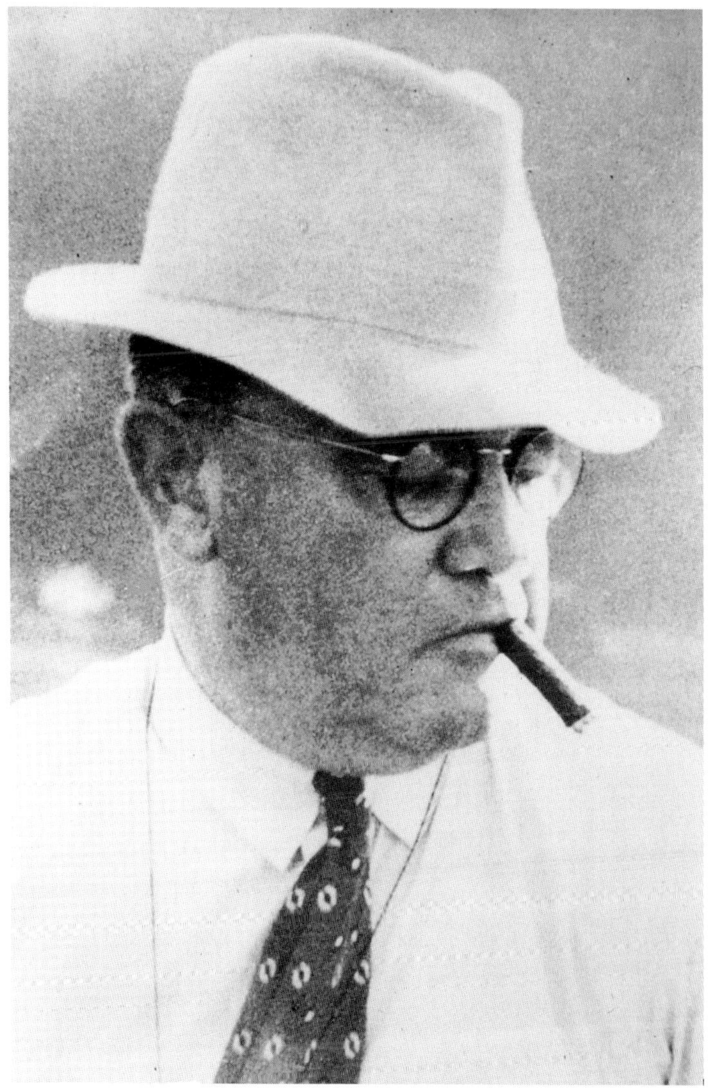

*Walther Straub*

# Walther Straub
## 1874 – 1944 *

Walther Straub was born at Augsburg on May 18, 1874. His father was a lawyer and later became an official of the State of Bavaria. In 1892 W. Straub began the study of medicine at München University, then spent some time at Tübingen University and completed his clinical studies at Strassburg in 1897. As a medical student he already had done some experimental work under O. Schmiedeberg on glycosuria during poisoning with carbon monoxide which was published (Straub, 1897). He completed his medical studies in München University where he received his degree of Dr.med. on July 18, 1897, for which he presented a further publication based on experimental work (Straub, 1899). At the same time he entered the Department of Physiology at the University of München as an Assistant under Carl Voit. One of the memorable events of this period was Straub's acquaintance with his life-long friend, Otto Frank. Frank had already been in Voit's laboratory since 1894 and became famous through his work "Zur Dynamik des Herzmuskels", which, in 1905, he presented as part of the requirement for qualification as a Lecturer in Physiology (on the life of O. Frank, see Wezler, 1950).

Straub's career as a pharmacologist started in 1898 when he entered the laboratories of pharmacology at Leipzig University as an Assistant to Rudolf Boehm. Already on July 23, 1900 he qualified as a Lecturer in Pharmacology. During the Leipzig period he visited the Zoological Station at Naples, Italy, where he had an opportunity to use marine animals for physiological and pharmacological studies. Not yet a full professor, Straub in

---

* Biographical sources: Bock, 1971; Forst, 1974; Haffner, 1944; Heubner, 1944; Lindner, 1957; Rost, 1947; Stroomann, 1960.

1905 assumed the direction of the Department of Pharmacology at the University of Marburg and relinquished this position after less than a year when he was called to the University of Würzburg as Professor of Pharmacology and head of the department. A year and a half later he moved to the University of Freiburg i.Br. where he remained from 1907 to 1923 and was given the opportunity to erect a new building with modern facilities for research and teaching in pharmacology and toxicology. In 1923 Straub followed a call to the University of München as Professor of Pharmacology and Toxicology. As at Freiburg he took upon himself the task of transforming this department into an exemplary place for the scientific and educational tasks of pharmacology and toxicology. He guided the work of this department until he became emeritus professor early in 1944, only shortly before his death in Bad Tölz on October 22, 1944.

In 1900, when Straub started his academic career as a Lecturer in Pharmacology, the characteristic pharmacological effects of a large number of drugs were established. However, the description centered entirely on the qualitative nature of the physiological alterations; quantitative considerations were just beginning to receive attention. It was the transition from qualitative to the quantitative aspects of drug action in which Straub took a leading part. Moreover, he was interested in the chemical fate of the drug on the way to the site of action as well as in the whole complex of biological events from the site of action to the changes in the responding organ which, in the normal organism, are responsible for the physiological effect and, in the diseased organism, for the therapeutic effect.

Also, with regard to the type of drugs, Straub's interests were broad. He and his pupils dealt with drugs of many different groups and, depending upon the requirements of the problem, the methods were chemical, physical, or biological. Of greatest importance for the study of the quantitative aspects of drug action were the investigations on isolated organs, or parts of organ systems, which Straub either invented or which he and his pupils used extensively and further developed, e.g., the isolated frog heart that bears Straub's name, the perfused preparation of the hindlegs of the frog, first used by Fraser (1892) and developed for quantitative measurements by P. Trendelenburg, the preparation of the isolated small intestine first described by R. Magnus. Such preparations made it possible to investigate drugs directly at the organ containing the site of action, independently of the influences of the organism as a whole. In addition, these relatively simple preparations and their quantitative responses to alterations in dose or concentration of active agents provided the investigator with methods (tools) to achieve two important aims: 1) at a time when chemical or physical methods were not yet available, it became possible to ascertain the presence of minute amounts of a substance (drug, active principle) in biological systems; and 2) the methods were useful in assessing by bioassay the value – claimed and often wanting – of therapeutic agents or preparations.

At the turn of the century little thought was given to problems of general pharmacology. Straub recognized clearly the paramount importance of these problems for the establishment of the foundation of pharmacology as a biological science. Boehm (see for instance, 1895) already had given thought to general problems of pharmacology, e.g., selectivity of drug action, absorption, distribution and degradation in the organism, changes of concentration at the site of action; but his pupils Heffter and Straub were the first to begin the experimental investigation of these problems. As Straub (1903) put it himself, he provided for Boehm's thoughts "ziffernmäßige Unterlagen", i. e., the underpinning with figures, the experimentally obtained quantitative data.

Using the isolated heart of the sea snail, Aplysia limacina, Straub (1903) carried out quantitative studies with veratrine hydrochloride, curarine, and strychnine. With these alkaloids or alkaloid mixtures he found accumulation in the cardiac tissue. On the basis of the data he devoloped his concepts on accumulation of a substance in body tissue, diffusion through cell membranes, specific activity, degradation, equilibrium between tissue concentration and concentration in the solution outside the tissue. In this paper the principle of bioassay is clearly stated and illustrated by the three biological systems selected by Straub for quantitative evaluation.

Similarly and very early Straub (1907) gave consideration to the problem of drug antagonism especially in connection with the kinetics of the action of muscarine and the muscarine-atropine antagonism. In this series of investigations he developed the controversial concept that with certain substances, e.g. muscarine, the concentration change during the penetration into the cell may be decisive for the biological effect.

Throughout his scientific career, Straub devoted much attention to the action of the digitalis substances. In contrast to the alkaloids he found no accumulation of these substances in the tissue of the isolated heart of the cold blooded animals and concluded that, for the biological effect of this group of substances, a physicochemical process of fixation to the cell membrane and a disturbance of its exchange function may be of fundamental importance. To clarify the chemism of the reaction Straub attempted to determine the dose that must be bound to the heart muscle in order to obtain a definite reaction (e. g., tonic standstill). Since extraction of the ventricle proved unsuccessful, because there was no accumulation, Straub developed a difference or use-up method to determine the consumption of the digitalis glycoside (Straub, 1910). Transfer of an exact amount of the filling fluid after completion of the biological reaction from the first to a second heart, then from the second to a third etc. heart, made it possible to calculate the decrease in concentration in the filling fluid, and, respectively, the amount of the glycoside for the characteristic biological reaction (e.g., tonic standstill) of one heart. For these experimental conditions Straub (1924, pp. 1370–1571) recognized the dependence of the glycoside effect upon concentration. Moreover, this type of experiment led to the finding that, in the isolated heart of the frog (Rana esculenta), the effect of the digitalis glycosides is preceded by a latency period wich cannot be shortened by very high concentrations (e. g., 11 min; P. Trendelenburg, 1909). Straub's pupil, P. Trendelenburg, concluded that the mechanism of the cardiac glycoside effect is biphasic: the physiological final effect which can be recorded is preceded by a physiologically latent chemical action.

An outgrowth of these early experimental studies of Straub and his pupils was his intense interest in the role of the cell membrane for pharmacological activity ("für pharmakologisches Geschehen"). In a lecture to biologists and physicians Straub (1912a) spoke of the importance of the cell membrane ("als die erste Etappe auf dem Weg zur Erklärung der Spezifität der Wirkung chemischer Stoffe im Organismus") as the first step on the way to an explanation of the specificity of the action of chemical compounds in the organism. He pointed to the difficulties of a rational synthesis of specific (selective) remedies and said: with every influence to be exerted upon the living organism the cell membrane has to be taken into account. It is "ein Zellularorgan", an organ of the cell which is different from cell to cell, and in the same cell it may be altered from moment to moment. Poignantly, he stressed: every active substance must go to the cell membrane, into the cell membrane, or through the cell membrane; and each one of these deformations of the cell membrane may be the sole cause of a change in function, i.e., of a pharmacological action.

With his pupil, H. Weese, Straub extended his investigations on the fate of the digitalis glycosides to the organism of the cat. In the meantime the chemical nature, e.g., of digitoxin and g-strophanthin (ouabain), had been elucidated. Their lethal doses were determined in the cat heart using Starling's heart-lung preparation. The amount used up by other organs, e.g. kidney, liver, skeletal muscle, lung, was found by inserting them into the heart-lung circuit and determining the increased (or, in case of the lung, unchanged) lethal dose for the heart. The results of such experiments provided Straub with the data for his concept of the ("Effektivdosis") effective dose of the digitalis substances (Straub, 1929, 1931b) and for the theory of the digitalis effect (Straub, 1932). Even today it is a very stimulating experience to follow Straub's thoughts on this matter although the analytical data on distribution, degradation and excretion of the digitalis substances obtained by modern chemical and physicochemical methods led to extensive revision of the findings of Straub and Wecse.

Of lasting value are Straub's fundamental studies on the change by the digitalis glycosides of the contraction of the cardiac muscle. He was the first (Straub, 1905) to apply the principles established by his friend Otto Frank to the investigation of the non-lethal cardiac effect. On the excised ventricle of the frog heart with exact volumetric recording Straub measured the pulse volume of single contractions at constant initial tension. At the beginning of the digitalis effect the pulse volume was increased. At this stage there also was an increase above the normal values of the tension curve of the isometric maxima. The two observations led to the conclusion, similar to that derived by Boehm (1872) from experiments at the frog heart with the Ludwig-Coats method (Coats, 1869), that, provided there is enough fluid to be moved by the heart, the cardiac work of the individual heat will be increased by digitalis (Straub, 1924, p. 1428).

Likewise, in the intact circulation of the cat, Straub (1908) made a decisive contribution to our knowledge of the fundamental cardiac effects of the digitalis substances. He examined the form of the intraventricular pressure curves of the left ventricle, using a troikart manometer of fairly high frequency. To prevent interference with blood flow and with the cardiac valves, the manometer was placed into the left ventricle through the apex of the heart. It was found that ouabain in therapeutic doses made the ascending limb of the contraction curve steeper (increased the rate of contraction), shortened the time of contraction ("Anspannungszeit war verkürzt"), and blood volume was expelled with greater velocity by the ventricle. Straub's intellectual and experimental part at the beginning of the elucidation of the circulatory action of the digitalis substances is best seen in his literary contribution "Die Digitalisgruppe" in which he critically reviewed the older literature up to the year 1914 (see especially Straub, 1924, Chapter III., pp. 1394–1452).

Straub had a great interest in physiological processes and in comparative physiological considerations. The investigation of the circulation of Aplysia limacina is a good example of this. As mentioned above, he used the isolated working cardiac muscle for the study of the accumulation of various alkaloids. However, the use of this organ was not limited to serving as a test object; rather, he subjected the heart and circulation to a thorough physiological investigation (Straub, 1904). In the aplysia heart, using an elegant method of his own, Straub, following the concepts of Otto Frank, studied the relationship between initial tension and pulse volume as well as the isometric activity of the ventricle muscle, as had Frank done in the frog heart. The circulatory system as a whole aroused Straub's interest, because it functions in a way entirely different from the system of the vertebrate animals. In aplysia the blood flows from the heart into the lacunes and into the body cavity, from there to the gills which are located outside the skin-muscle tube, and thence back into the atrium and ventricle of the heart. Straub found the innervation of the circulatory system to extend only to the gills, and the ventricle of the heart to be devoid of regulatory innervation. Hence, each contraction of the skin-muscle tube increases the inside pressure and leads to a greater flow of blood to the gills and on to the heart. As a result, the heart becomes heavily overloaded and responds with increase in pulse volume and frequency. Straub concluded that

it may be an exclusive property of the smooth cardiac musculature to start becoming rhythmically active on stretching and, if
stretching increases further, to accelerate the rhythm. He considered this "barynogenic" polyrhythmia (Tschermak, 1902, see
pp. 232–233) to be a general physiological principle.

The physiology of smooth muscle organs held great interest for
Straub. For example, the phenomenon of tonicity in invertebrates
occupied his thoughts (see Straub, 1901, p. 524) in his paper on
the aplysia heart where he says:"Tonicity of the contractile
organs is of great physiological importance for invertebrate animals. Presumably because the tonicity of the muscle cell plays
the role of the skeleton by determining the length and the effective range of the muscle, in the same way as is done by the length
of the bone between the two attachments of the striated muscles
in the vertebrate animals."

In this field of the physiology and pharmacology of the tubular
organs Straub, towards the end of his career, achieved one more
great success as an active investigator in the natural sciences.
Shortly after the death, in 1931, of his pupil Paul Trendelenburg,
he took up the latter's studies on intestinal motility (Trendelenburg, P., 1913, 1917). Trendelenburg had used isolated segments
of guinea-pig small intestine proximally tied and with a cannula
inserted into the distal end, and which, in vitro, were exposed to
pressure changes from the inside in order to elicit peristaltic
movements. Straub developed this method for use in situ. This is
to say, the selected piece of gut retained its natural vascular and
nervous connections with the organism (Straub and Viaud, 1932).
Experiments were also carried out on segments of the large intestine (Straub and Schild, 1932). The tension curve of various segments of the small and large intestine was established by measuring the relationship between filling pressure and intestinal
volume; and the absorption of water, and of water from salt solutions was examined quantitatively (Straub and Leo, 1932, 1933;
Leo, 1933). The data served as a foundation for the analysis of

the action of various solanaceae and opium alkaloids, i.e., the atropine series (Straub and Munoz Fernandes, 1933) and the morphine series (Straub and Ozaki, 1933).

In the guinea-pig intestine atropine and l-hyoscyamine paralysed tonicity of the small intestine, while scopolamine had a marked paralysing effect on the large intestine. These alkaloids did not influence peristalsis. All opium alkaloids decreased tonicity of the small and large intestine. Morphine was most effective, papaverine least. None of the opium alkaloids paralysed peristalsis. Lack of peristaltic activity is the indirect result of decrease in tone and due to deficient filling. The intestinal effect of opium is due entirely to the morphine it contains.

In order to approach more closely the conditions of the human gut, experiments were extended to the cat intestine with its larger musculature. The segment of the small, or large, intestine was provided with cannulae at both ends and, thus, as under physiological conditions, was able to perform peristaltic transport work. By measuring inflow and outflow of fluid absorption also could be assessed quantitatively (Straub and Triendl, 1934a). The most important pharmacological result of these studies was the analysis of the activity of Folia Sennae (Straub and Triendl, 1934b). It led to the elucidation of the site of action and of the nature of the active principles (Straub and Triendl, 1937).

The therapeutically valuable action of the Senna glycosides is a stimulation of the large intestine without influence on pendular movements. After oral administration of threshold doses (in man!) the active substances are completely absorbed in the small intestine and transported via the blood stream to the site of action. There is a characteristic latency period lasting several hours between the oral intake and the effect. During this time the active substances, easily absorbed as glycosides, are chemically altered by enzymatic cleavage of anthranol and its oxidation to anthrachinone. The latter probably is the active principle.

Straub was a great teacher. His presentation was vivid and exciting and on occasion full of humour and worldly wisdom. He had a sovereign command of his subject and was a master of the word. It was Straub's conviction that, in the natural sciences part of medicine, the experiment was of paramount importance. "The facts of the natural sciences and especially of the experimental sciences", he said, "are facts of experience"; "man muß sie erleben" (one has to witness them). Straub's lectures were prepared with great care. With his artistic sense (he was a great photographer and amateur painter) and his great skill and vast experience as an experimenter he devised many novel lecture demonstrations. They employed simple means, could be easily understood and were often very beautiful (Stroomann, 1960). For many of his listeners, some of Straub's demonstrations of physiological processes or drug actions (Straub, 1912b) were unforgettable events. Frequently he enlivened his formal presentations on drugs and poisons by references to historical events. Some of these remarks were based on literary studies which have been preserved (e.g., Über Genußgifte, Straub, 1926; Der Tod Alexanders VI. und das Borgia-Geheimnis, Straub, 1935; Phosphor, Straub, 1944).

# *References*

BOCK, R. (1971). Personalbibliographien von Professoren und Dozenten der Hygiene und Pharmakologie an der Med. Fak. d. Univ. Würzburg im ungefähren Zeitraum von 1900-1945. Inaugural-Diss., Erlangen Nürnberg.

BOEHM, R. (1872). Untersuchungen über die physiologische Wirkung der Digitalis und des Digitalin. Pflügers Arch. ges. Physiol., 5, 153 191.

BOEHM, R. (1895). Einige Bemerkungen über die Nervenendwirkung des Curarin. Arch. exp. Path. Pharmakol., 35, 16-22.

COATS, J. (1869). Wie ändern sich durch die Erregung des n. vagus die Arbeit und die innern Reize des Herzens? Aus dem physiologischen Institute zu Leipzig. Vorgelegt von dem wirklichen Mitgliede Prof. C. Ludwig. Ber. Königl.-Sächs. Akad. d. Wissensch., 21, 360-391.

FORST, A. W. (1974). Walther Straub 100 Jahre. Münch. med. Wschr., 116, 1171-1174.

FRASER, Th. R. (1892). Strophanthus hispidus: its natural history, chemistry and pharmacology. Pharmacology: Trans. Roy. Soc. Edinburgh, 36, II, 343-457.

HAFFNER, F. (1944). An Walther Straub. Münch. med. Wschr., 91, 343-344.

HEUBNER, W. (1944). Zu Walther Straubs 70. Geburtstag (8. Mai 1944). Klin. Wschr., 23, 139-140.

LEO, E. (1933). Studien über Darmmotilität IV. Zur Physiologie und Pharmakologie der Dünndarmperistaltik. Arch. exp. Path. Pharmakol., 169, 25-33.

LINDNER, J. (1957). Zeittafeln zur Geschichte der pharmakologischen Institute des deutschen Sprachgebietes. Aulendorf i. Württ.: Editio Cantor.

ROST, E. (1947). Walther Straub in memoriam! Med.Klin., 42, 202-204.

STRAUB, W. (1897). Über die Bedingungen des Auftretens der Glykosurie nach Kohlenoxydvergiftung. Arch. exp. Path. Pharmak., 38, 139-157.

STRAUB, W. (1899). Über den Einfluß des Kochsalzes auf die Eiweißzersetzung. Z. Biol., 37, 527-549.

STRAUB, W. (1901). Zur Physiologie des Aplysienherzens. Pflügers Arch. ges. Physiol., 86, 504-532.

STRAUB, W. (1903). Quantitative Untersuchungen über das Eindringen von Alkaloiden in lebende Zellen. Pflügers Arch. ges. Physiol., 98, 233-240.

STRAUB, W. (1904). Fortgesetzte Studien am Aplysienherzen (Dynamik, Kreislauf und dessen Innervation) nebst Bemerkungen zur vergleichenden Muskelphysiologie. Pflügers Arch. ges. Physiol., 103, 429-449.

STRAUB, W. (1905). Dynamik des Froschherzventrikels bei nicht tödlicher Digitalisvergiftung. Z. exp. Path. Ther., 1, 489-512.

STRAUB, W. (1907). Zur chemischen Kinetik der Muskarinwirkung und des Antagonismus Muskarin-Atropin. Pflügers Arch. ges. Physiol., 119, 127-151.

STRAUB, W. (1908). Die Elementarwirkung der Digitaliskörper. Sitzungsber. d. Physikal.-med. Gesellschaft Würzburg, Jg. 1907, 85-93.

STRAUB, W. (1910). Quantitative Untersuchungen über den Chemismus der Strophanthinwirkung. Biochem. Z., 28, 392-407.

STRAUB, W. (1912a). Die Bedeutung der Zellmembran für die Wirkung chemischer Stoffe im Organismus. Naturw. Rdsch. (Braunschweig), 27, 621-624; 639-642; 649-652.

STRAUB, W. (1912b). Vorlesungsversuche zur Theorie der Narkose. Z. biol. Technik u. Methodik, 2, 277-279.

STRAUB, W. (1920). Naturwissenschaften und Pharmakologie im Medizinischen Unterricht. Dtsch. med. Wschr., 46, 246-247; 270-271; 300-301.

STRAUB, W. (1924). Die Digitalisgruppe. In Heffters Handb. exp. Pharmakol., 2, Teil II, 1355-1452. Berlin: Springer.

STRAUB, W. (1926). Über Genußgifte. Naturwissenschaften, 14, 1091-1099.

STRAUB, W. (1929).Neuere Digitalisforschung. In: Pathologie und Therapie der Zirkulationsstörungen. VI. Fortbildungslehrgang in Bad Nauheim 18.-20. Sept., 33-41. Leipzig: Thieme.

STRAUB, W. (1931a). Paul Trendelenburg †. Dtsch. med. Wschr., 57, 374-376.

STRAUB, W. (1931b). Die Effektivdosis der Digitalisstoffe. Z. ärztl. Fortbild., 28, 1-3.

STRAUB, W. (1932). Bau, Resorption und Bindung der Digitalisstoffe. In Der Weg zur rationellen Therapie, Vorträge: Heidelberg 1.-3. August 1932, 46-56. Leipzig:Thieme.

STRAUB, W. (1935). Der Tod Alexanders VI. und das Borgia-Geheimnis. Schweiz. med. Wschr., 65, 389-392.

STRAUB, W. (1944). Phosphor. Straßburger Monatshefte, 8, 54-56.

STRAUB, W. & LEO, E. (1932). Studien zur Darmmotilität III. Der Tonus und die Dehnungskurve des ruhenden Darmes. Arch. exp. Path. Pharmakol., 169, 18-24.

STRAUB, W. & LEO, E. (1933). Resorption von Wasser und von Wasser aus Salzlösungen im Darm. Arch. exp. Path. Pharmak., 170, 534-545.

STRAUB, W. & MUNOZ FERNANDES, E. (1933). Studien über Darmmotilität V. Totalanalyse der Alkaloide der Atropingruppe. Arch. exp. Path. Pharmakol., 170, 26-38.

STRAUB, W. & OZAKI, M. (1933). Studien über Darmmotilität VI. Totalanalyse der Alkaloide der Morphingruppe. Arch. exp. Path. Pharmakol., 173, 374-380.

STRAUB, W. & SCHILD, H. (1932). Über Darmmotilität II. Zur Physiologie und Pharmakologie des Dickdarmes. Arch. exp. Path. Pharmakol., 169, 9-17.

STRAUB, W. & TRIENDL, E. (1934a). Peristaltik und Wasserresorption im Katzendarm. Arch. exp. Path. Pharmakol., 175, 518-527.

STRAUB, W. & TRIENDL, E. (1934b). Über die Wirkung des Senna-Infuses auf den Dickdarm der Katze. Arch. exp. Path. Pharmakol., 175, 528-535.

STRAUB, W. & TRIENDL, E. (1937). Theorie der Abführwirkung der Folia Sennae und ihrer wirksamen Inhaltsstoffe. Arch. exp. Path. Pharmakol., 185, 1-19.

STRAUB, W. & VIAUD, P. (1932). Über Darmmotilität I. Methodik. Arch. exp. Path. Pharmakol., 169, 1-8.

STROOMANN, G. (1960). Aus meinem Roten Notizbuch. 2.Aufl., Frankfurt/Main: Societätsverlag.

TRENDELENBURG, P. (1909). Vergleichende Untersuchungen über den Wirkungsmechanismus und die Wirkungsintensität glykositischer Herzgifte. Arch. exp. Path. Pharmakol., 61, 256-273.

TRENDELENBURG, P. (1913). Eine neue Methode zur Registrierung der Darmtätigkeit. Z. Biol., 61, 67-72.

TRENDELENBURG, P. (1917). Physiologische und pharmakologische Versuche über die Dünndarmperistaltik. Arch. exp. Path. Pharmakol., 81, 57-129.

TSCHERMAK, A. (1902). Über den Einfluß lokaler Belastung auf die Leistungsfähigkeit des Skeletmuskels. Pflügers Arch. ges. Physiol., 91, 217-247.

WEZLER, K. (1950). O. Frank zum Gedächtnis. Z. Biol., 103, 91-122.

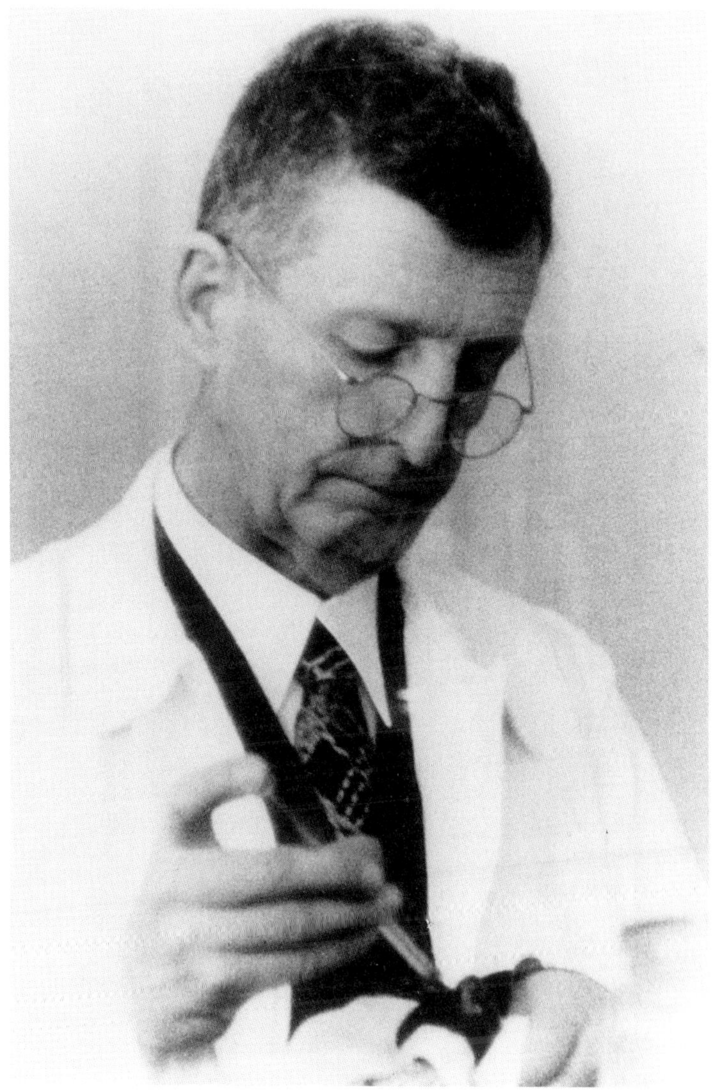

*Oscar Gros*

# Oscar Gros
## 1877 – 1947[*]

Franz Jakob Oscar Gros was born on March 13, 1877 in Werneck near Würzburg, where his father, Peter Gros, was a general practitioner. After having finished school in Würzburg he read chemistry, first at that city's university from 1896 to 1898 and then at Leipzig, where, in March 1901, he obtained his Dr. phil. with the thesis "On the sensitivity to light of fluorethin, its substituted derivatives and their leukobases" (Gros, 1901). He was then assistant at the Mining Academy in Clausthal for six months and subsequently, for 18 months, at the Department of Physical Chemistry of the University of Leipzig under Wilhelm Ostwald.

Subsequently Gros read medicine in Leipzig from 1903 to 1908. During the last three years of his medical studies he was assistant in the Department of Pharmacology under Rudolf Boehm. In 1908 he obtained the degree of Dr. med., with the thesis "Observations on the action of curarine in rabbits with special considerations of the time course of detoxication and the claimed antagonism between curarine and physostigmine" (Gros, 1908). One year later he was inducted as Lecturer in Pharmacology under Boehm with the thesis "Studies on haemolysis" (Gros, 1909). At the beginning of 1915 he received the title of Professor. In September of the same year he was offered the chair of pharmacology in Halle, as the successor to Erich Harnack. After his appointment "the militia member Professor Gros was assigned, as a physician, to the Prussian military administration at Halle" with permission granted to carry out academic teaching. Until the end of the First World War Gros was repeatedly

---

[*] Biographical sources: Gelbke, 1956; Lindner, 1957; Lendle, 1966; Poggendorff, 1904; 1937; 1957; Kroker-Wawrzinek, 1977.

ordered to work at the Kaiser-Wilhelm-Institute for Physical Chemistry in Berlin-Dahlem. After the war, at the end of 1919, he accepted the first chair of pharmacology at the newly founded University of Köln, but, soon, in 1922 moved to the University of Kiel. Although his predecessor August Falck had directed this department as an "extraordinary professor", Gros was offered the position of full professor; thereby raising the status of pharmacology in Kiel to that of other German universities. He was also asked to teach pharmacognosy. In 1925 he returned to Leipzig, to accept Boehm's old chair as the successor of Fühner. At the beginning of the Second World War he was again drafted into the army. In 1942 he asked for early retirement, which was granted in March 1943. His pupil Ludwig Lendle came from Münster as his successor. Gros spent his last years in Uffing on the Staffelsee, where he died on August 3, 1947.

Gros was greatly influenced by having worked in physical chemistry under Wilhelm Ostwald. His physical and chemical knowledge obviously made him an appreciated co-worker of Rudolf Boehm. The physicochemical approach influenced his own research, such as his "Studies on haemolysis" (Gros, 1907a,b, 1909, 1910d,e). Since the temperature coefficient of haemolysis was much greater than that of the formation of methaemoglobin from the haemoglobin released by haemolysis, he was able to measure colorimetrically the time course of haemolysis at higher temperatures. Using this method he carried out his fundamental studies on the haemolytic activity of isotonic solutions of alkaline salts, which seemingly do not damage red blood cells at physiological temperature. Since at this temperature haemolysis proceeds far too slowly to allow exact measurements, he used temperatures of 47.5 °C, 50.0 °C and 52.5 °C to compare the haemolytic effects of isotonic solutions of the chlorides of sodium, potassium, magnesium and calcium as well as the sulphates of sodium, potassium and magnesium. He observed pronounced differences between the haemolysis-inducing effects of the different salts and their ions. An exception was magnesium ion

(Gros, 1909), the action of which could be regarded as protective. On the other hand, the strong haemolytic activities of ammonia, sodium carbonate and sodium hydroxide were studied at physiological temperature (37.5 °C); kinetic differences were explained by their different dissociation constants (Gros, 1910d,e).

With respect to the bactericidal effect of silver compounds, Gros investigated the physicochemical properties of colloidal precious metals and their pharmacological effects (Gros and O'Connor, 1911), and especially the mechanism of action of colloidal silver halogenides (Gros, 1911; 1912a,d).

In an extensive series of publications "On general and local anaesthetics", Gros investigated the relationship between these two groups of substances. For local anaesthetics he found a high oil : water partition coefficient and also that they were able to cause full anaesthesia in frogs through an action on the central nervous system. The latter was much more sensitive to general anaesthetics than the peripheral nervous system. Thus, certain water-soluble general anaesthetics were relatively weak local anaesthetics. However, he failed "to find any clues justifying a theoretical mechanistic separation of general and local anaesthetics" (Gros, 1910a, b; Gros and Hartung, 1910). Of practical importance was his observation that the free bases of local anaesthetics exerted their effects more quickly than their salts and were more potent. The addition of sodium bicarbonate to a solution of procaine [Novocain®] hydrochloride increased by hydrolysis the concentration of the free base, and thereby its local anaesthetic effect (Gros, 1910b,c). This enhancement of local anaesthetic activity, demonstrated in animal experiments, was confirmed in patients by Straub's pupil A. Laewen at the Surgical University Hospital of Leipzig under Friedrich Trendelenburg. "In man, solutions of Novocain® bicarbonate are effective on sensory nerve endings in concentrations which are two- to three-fold lower than those of Novocain hydrochloride" (Laewen, 1910). Additional studies concerned the stability of free bases of local anaesthetics in solutions and the effects of various salts of procaine (Gros, 1912b,c). In experiments with the nerve-muscle preparation of the frog he, together with Kochmann, found that the inhibition of nerve conduction by procaine chloride solutions is accelerated by the addition of potassium salts (Gros and Kochmann, 1923). Later on Gros investigated the antagonism between general anaesthetics and pentylenetetrazol [Cardiazol®] and nikethamide [Coramin®] (Gros, 1936; Gros and Haas, 1936) as well as the effectiveness of a combination of pentylenetetrazol and ephedrine in barbitone [Veronal®] intoxication (Gros and Hofmann, 1936).

The scientific publications of Gros stemmed mainly from his stay in the Leipzig department under Bochm. The war and Gros's frequent changes of universities may well have contributed to his subsequently not having been overly productive either experimentally or literarily. Moreover, Gros himself was not inclined towards the formulation of theories; this appears to have prevented him from demonstrating the importance of physicochemical concepts for general pharmacology. Typical of Gros's relation to his assistants and coworkers is a letter written in 1942, shortly before his retirement. He wrote to a former pupil: "You know well that my assistants have total freedom in the choice of their area of research, as soon as they have become proficient and I have convinced myself of their aptitude; my own contribution is then restricted to occasional proposals and suggestions. I am convinced that this optimally advances the self confidence, the interest in, and the enjoyment of, their work, which is then the assistant's own spiritual property. It is possible that the criticism which I offer after completion of the study is occasionally regarded as exaggerated or painful. However, I regard especially rigorous criticism as necessary, since it results in the most important contribution to the assistant's training and further career, namely the need to ensure the complete reliability of the results and the most critical possible examination of the conclusions."

As an academic teacher of medical students, he especially emphasized subjects like general and local anaesthesia, expectorants and the pharmacology of inorganic compounds. Following the tradition of Boehm and Fühner, he paid special attention to the teaching of pharmacy students, including giving lectures on pharmacognosy and providing a pharmacognosy course.

# *References*

GELBKE, N. (1956). Die geschichtliche Entwicklung des Pharmakologischen Instituts der Leipziger Universität unter besonderer Berücksichtigung der Gründerjahre. Inaugural-Diss., Leipzig.

GROS, O. (1901). Über die Lichtempfindlichkeit des Fluorethins, seine substituierten Derivate, sowie der Leukobasen derselben. Diss.phil., Leipzig. Z. physik. Chemie, 37, 1901.

GROS, O. (1907a). Über das Auftreten der Lackfarbe in Blutkörperchensuspensionen unter dem Einflusse der Wärme. 1. Mitteilung. Arch. exp. Path. Pharmakol., 57, 64-78.

GROS, O. (1907b). Über das Auftreten der Lackfarbe in Blutkörperchensuspensionen unter dem Einflusse der Wärme. 2. Mitteilung. Arch. exp. Path. Pharmakol., 57, 415-422.

GROS, O. (1908). Versuche über die Curarinwirkung bei Kaninchen mit besonderer Berücksichtigung des Entgiftungsverlaufes und des angeblichen Antagonismus zwischen Curarin und Physostigmin. Diss. med., Leipzig.

GROS, O. (1909). Studien über die Hämolyse. Habil.-Schrift, Leipzig. – Arch. exp. Path. Pharmakol., 62, 1-38.

GROS, O. (1910a). Über Narkotika und Lokalanästhetika. 1. Mitteilung Arch. exp. Path. Pharmakol., 62, 380-408.

GROS, O. (1910b). Über Narkotika und Lokalanästhetika. 2. Mitteilung. Arch.exp. Path. Pharmakol., 63, 80-106.

GROS, O. (1910c). Über eine Methode, die anästhesierende Wirkung der Lokalanästhetika zu steigern. Münchener med. Wschr., 57, 2042-2044.

GROS, O. (1910d). Studien über die Hämolyse. 2. Mitteilung. Die Hämolyse durch Natriumkarbonat. Arch. exp. Path. Pharmakol., 63, 341-346.

GROS, O. (1910e). Über die Hämolyse durch Ammoniak, Natriumhydroxyd und Natriumcarbonat. Biochem. Ztschr., 29, 350-367.

GROS, O. (1911). Über den Vorgang der bakteriziden Wirkung der Silberpräparate in kochsalzhaltigen Medien. Münchener med. Wschr., 58, 2659-2662.

GROS, O. (1912a). Über den Vorgang der bakteriziden Wirkung der Silberpräparate in kochsalzhaltigen Medien. 2. Mitteilung. Münchener med. Wschr., 59, 405-408.

GROS, O. (1912b). Über Narkotika und Lokalanästhetika 3. Mitteilung. Über die Beständigkeit der Basen der Lokalanästhetika in Lösung. Arch. exp. Path. Pharmakol., 67, 126-131.

GROS, O. (1912c). Über Narkotika und Lokalanästhetika. 4. Mitteilung. Über die Wirkung verschiedener Novokainsalze. Arch. exp. Path. Pharmakol., 67,132-136.

GROS, O. (1912d). Über den Wirkungsmechanismus kolloidaler Silberhalogenide. Arch. exp. Path. Pharmakol., 70, 375-406.

GROS, O. (1936). Beitrag zum gegenseitigen Antagonismus zwischen Cardiazol, Coramin und Narkotica. Arch. exp. Path. Pharmakol., 180, 258-265.

GROS, O. & HAAS, H. T. A. (1936). Der Antagonismus der Narkotica gegen Cardiazol. Arch. exp. Path. Pharmakol., 182, 348-362.

GROS, O. & HARTUNG, C. (1910). Über Narkotika und Lokalanästhetika. Nachtrag zur 2. Mitteilung. Arch. exp. Path. Pharmakol., 64, 67-71.

GROS, O. & HOFMANN, H. (1936). Über die Wirkung von Cardiazol, Ephedrin und der Kombination von Cardiazol und Ephedrin bei Veronalvergiftung. Klin. Wschr., 15, 1340-1341.

GROS, O. & KOCHMANN, M. (1923). Über einen neuen Mechanismus der potenzierenden Wirkung von Arzneigemischen unter besonderer Berücksichtigung von Novocain und Kaliumsulfat. Arch. exp. Path. Pharmakol., 98, 129-147.

GROS, O. & O`CONNOR, J. M. (1911). Einige Beobachtungen bei colloidalen Metallen mit Rücksicht auf ihre physikalisch-chemischen Eigenschaften. Arch. exp. Path. Pharmakol., 64, 456-467.

KROKER-WAWRZINEK, C. (1977). Die Entwicklung der Pharmakologie und des Pharmakologischen Institutes der Kieler Christiana Albertina (1855-1964). Inaugural-Diss., Kiel.

LAEWEN, A. (1910). Über die Verwendung des Novokains in Natriumbikarbonat-Kochsalzlösungen zur lokalen Anästhesie. Münchener med. Wschr., 57, 2044-2045.

LENDLE, L. (1966). Gros F. J. O. In: Neue deutsche Biographie, 7, 136-137. Berlin: Duncker & Humblot.

LINDNER, J. (1957). Zeittafeln zur Geschichte der pharmakologischen Institute des deutschen Sprachgebietes. Aulendorf i. Württ.: Editio Cantor.

POGGENDORFF, J. C. (1904). Gros, Oscar. Biogr.-Liter. Hdwrtb., IV; (1937) VI; (1957) VII a.

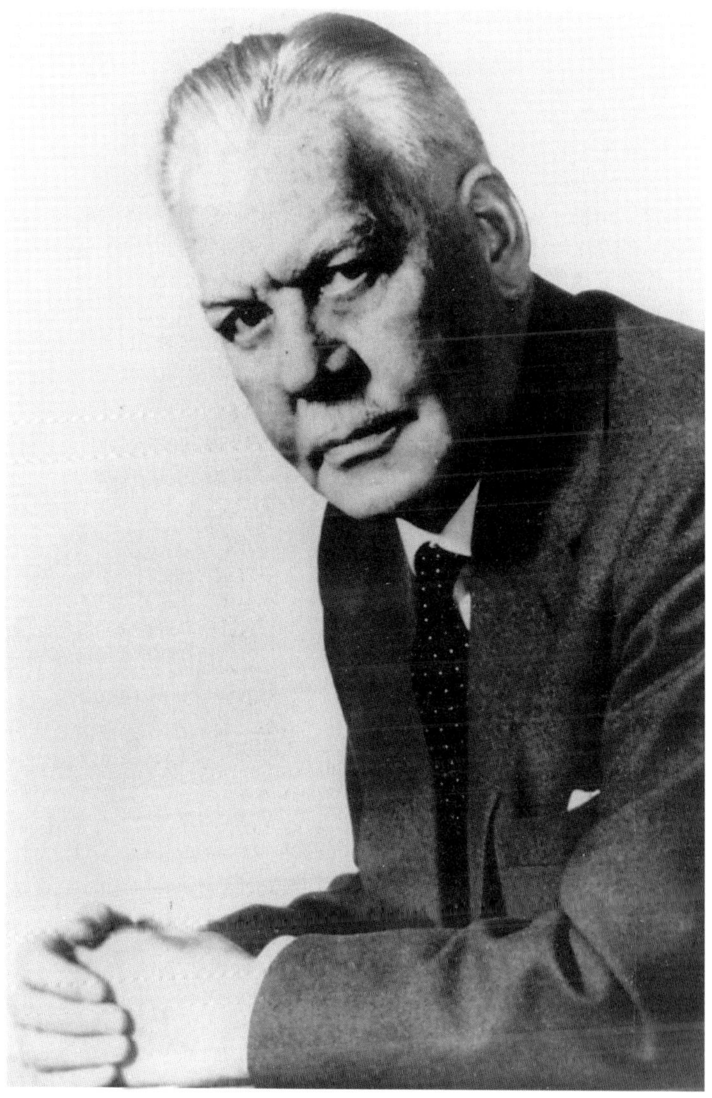

*Josef Schüller*

# Josef Schüller
# 1888 – 1968 *

Josef Schüller was born in Köln on February 21, 1888, the son of a merchant. After having attended the Kaiser-Wilhelm-Gymnasium in Köln he read chemistry and subsequently medicine, at the universities of Greifswald, Bonn and München. Under the supervision of R. Anschütz he received his Dr. phil. in Bonn in 1912, and in 1914 his Dr. med. under F. v. Müller in München, with the thesis "On the biological importance of acetylated compounds in the organism"; subsequently he was licenced as a physician. Throughout the First World War he served as a medical officer, despite being wounded in the first year of the war, with thereafter a bullet lodged permanently in his pericardium.

After the war Schüller joined Rudolf Boehm as an assistant in the Department of Pharmacology in Leipzig. There, in 1921 he qualified as a Lecturer in Pharmacology, with the thesis "On the physiological and pharmacological investigation of the frog rectum" (Schüller, 1921). In the same year – and after Boehm had retired – he moved to the University of Freiburg to join Walther Straub in the Department of Pharmacology. In 1922, at the age of 34 he was offered and accepted the directorship of the department in Köln, as successor to Oscar Gros. The university had been founded three years earlier, and the "Department" consisted of just two rooms located in a former fort, a remnant of the razed fortifications of the city. Schüller strove hard to obtain a building which offered adequate conditions for work. Eventually one became available in 1932. It consisted of a large, L-shaped former monastery building, the three floors of which offered 28

---

* Biographical sources: Corsten, 1938; Lindner, 1957; Poggendorff, 1960; Hamacher, 1970.

laboratories, a well stocked library and large rooms for practical courses in pharmacology, envisaged already at that time. The importance of these developments for Schüller can be deduced from the fact that he refused offers of chairs of pharmacology from the universities of Tübingen (1927), Göttingen (1929) and Heidelberg (1932). Towards the end of the Second World War his department was destroyed in one of the air raids. However, by 1948 the department was again functioning provisionally in the "balneology building" of the Hospital for Internal Medicine – equipped with apparatus, books and furniture that had been evacuated from Köln during the war. Schüller officially retired in 1956 but remained acting head until 1959. He died in Köln on September 12, 1968.

In his early studies in the Biological Laboratory of the University of Bonn, Schüller worked experimentally "on automatic centres and reflexes in the isolated intestine" of the frog with particular emphasis on the anatomical and functional particularities of the rectum (Schüller, 1911b). He described the existence of an automatic centre at the caudal end of the gastrointestinal tract which initiated periodic defecation movements when inhibitory influences from the spinal cord were removed. After the war these observations were extended in Boehm's department by investigations of the "isolated rectum preparation" developed by Schüller. It consisted of the distal part of the terminal gastrointestinal tract, which exhibited spontaneous rhythmic contractions. The contractions appeared to be maximal and were essentially analogous to those of cardiac muscle. As far as the pharmacology of the rectum preparation was concerned, it largely reflected that of other intestinal preparations (Schüller, 1921).

Even before his studies in Bonn, as a student of chemistry and medicine, Schüller had worked in the Department of Physiology of the Köln Academy for Practical Medicine. On the suggestion of its director, M. Cremer, Schüller carried out extensive "chemical and physiological studies on phloridzin", with the aim of clarifying its excretion from the organism. He succeeded in demonstrating that most of this diabetogenic substance was eliminated as a complex with glucuronic acid, named by him as phloridzin glucuronic acid. This paired acid contains not only the dextrose of phloridzin but also glucuronic acid bound like a glucoside. Animal experiments demonstrated that conjugation with glucuronic acid amounted to detoxication of phloridzin, since it resulted in a loss of diabetogenic action (Schüller, 1911a; see also Forst, pp. 476–477, 1966).

Various aspects of detoxication mechanisms occupied Schüller subsequently in Freiburg and Köln. Considering the fact that the chemical alteration of xenobiotics by "pairing" with sulphuric acid, glucuronic acid, glycocoll [glycine], glutamic acid etc. is associated with their detoxication, the question arose whether the biological process of detoxication was due to the same change in the physical or chemical properties of the xenobiotics. The chemically very different classes of paired substances have in common that they are readily soluble in water, while being virtually insoluble in "lipid" solvents; hence, their ether/water partition coefficients are very low. On the other hand, xenobiotics which are subject to "pairing", such as phenols, the camphor group, bromobenzol, benzoic acid and other aromatic acids, are characterized by a very high lipid solubility. If lipid soluble substances are conjugated with lipid insoluble components, the resulting molecules lose their lipid solubility and, hence, their ability to enter the lipid phase. "Thus, the essential effect of this pairing is a change in the distribution of the substance in the organism; lipid soluble, cytotropic, toxic substances are thus turned into lipid insoluble, nontoxic ones" (Schüller, 1925c).

If the transformation of lipid soluble substances (which easily penetrate into the cells) into lipid insoluble ones is the essential feature of this process, then one would expect that not all members of a group of substances would be subject to pairing, but only those characterized by a high partition coefficient. Schüller tested this hypothesis for conjugates of aromatic acids with glycine, also using relevant information from the literature. Comparison of a large number of aromatic acids with either low or high lipid solubilities revealed that in vivo "pairing" with glycine occured only for acids with an oil/water partition coefficient greater than 3 (Schüller, 1925c).

Schüller measured the demarcation potential of the muscle as an indicator of the entry of substances into the muscle cells. This potential develops between an injured and an intact region of the muscle as a function of the lipid solubility of the agents, the latter being positive versus the injured portion. Schüller started from the observation that the neutral salts of acids, consistent with their very poor lipid solubility, failed to induce such a potential, while the free acids, released from the salts by the addition of $CO_2$, increased the potential difference to a greater extent, the more lipid soluble they were. These results demonstrate a correlation between the lipid solubility of the substances, their ability to enter cells (as measured by the demarcation potential) and their tendency to complex with glycine (Schüller, 1923; 1925c; 1930).

Studies of the antagonism by local anaesthetics of either the "veratrine response" or the caffeine-induced muscle rigidity confronted Schüller with a different detoxication mechanism. The "veratrine response" consists of a characteristic protracted relaxation of a skeletal muscle contraction (see Boehm, 1920). Schüller and Athmer (1921) found it to be antagonized by various local anaesthetics, such as Novocain® [procaine] and Anesthesin® [benzocaine]; "in such a way that the initial twitch, which is more or less hidden in the veratrine curve, reappears unchanged" (Schüller and Athmer, 1921; Schüller, 1922a).

The caffeine-induced rigidity of the frog muscle was not reversed by procaine. In view of the destruction of the muscle – as seen under the microscope – this is not surprising. However, if the local anaesthetic is added simultaneously with caffeine – or if given as a pretreatment – "then a pronounced antagonism becomes evident: the muscle remains slack, retains its normal colour and shows no microscopic changes". Like procaine, benzocaine was also very effective (Schüller, 1922b, 1925b). Schüller obtained various indications that the antagonism of caffeine by the local anaesthetics is due to a chemical interaction: the complex-like binding of caffeine leads to loss of its activity. For instance, Schüller found the chloroform/water partition coefficient of caffeine to be reduced by the addition of increasing concentrations of procaine, while the addition of caffeine failed to lower the freezing point of a procaine solution (Schüller, 1925a).

According to this analysis the antagonism by procaine of the effect of caffeine on muscle is unrelated to the specific local anaesthetic action of procaine. The rank order of local anaesthetics for their physicochemical ability to form complexes corresponded to that for their ability to protect the muscle from caffeine-induced rigidity. Also other substances, lacking local anaesthetic activity, like sodium salicylate and sodium benzoate, were able to reduce or prevent caffeine-induced rigidity, by their ability to form complexes with caffeine. The ability of aequimolar concentrations of various substances to increase the solubility of caffeine, added in excess, served as a measure of their inclination to form such complexes. "The chemist may well be interested primarily in the question whether the resulting molecules have to be viewed as true complexes, as binding between different or identical molecules, or as simple aggregates, but this hardly affects the pharmacological conclusions" (Schüller, 1925a). For Schüller the biological phenomenon of alkaloid antagonism had progressed into the area of physicochemically analysable components. "The site of action involved a chemically defined substance, and the phenomenon interpreted as a true antagonism is in reality a pseudoantagonism" (Schüller, 1925a).

It was then of interest to him to test whether the antagonism between procaine and veratrine, described earlier (Schüller and

Athmer, 1921), is also of the caffeine type. Schüller found that veratrine base, which is poorly water soluble, dissolves easily in the presence of procaine; hence it resembles caffeine. This observation provided the explanation for the antagonism between procaine and veratrine as being due to a complex-like binding and consequent inactivation of veratrine by procaine. Further experiments demonstrated the abolition of the "veratrine response" by Na-salicylate, Na-cinnamylate and Na-Athophan® [cinchophen]. "The antagonism between the local anaesthetics and the aromatic salts tested here against the effects of caffeine and veratrine on the muscle involve the same principle. On the other hand, the processes underlying the antagonism of the local anaesthetics against contractures induced by excitatory substances (nicotine, choline, acetylcholine) must be of a different nature. No complex formation e.g., of procaine with choline or tetramethylammonium chloride could be demonstrated by determination of the freezing point" (Schüller, 1926).

Schüller's reports concerning the antagonism by procaine, sodium salicylate and sodium benzoate of the effect of caffeine on skeletal muscle, including their interpretation as a chemical event in the extracellular space, were confirmed by contemporary researchers (Zipf, 1930; Labes and Rutenbeck, 1933). However, in later studies of the antagonism against alkaloids in general, and especially that against the effect of veratrine on muscle, there was hardly any discussion of the importance of the formation of complex-like substances. This is the more remarkable, since pharmacists have become active after the Second World War, clarifying the binding mechanisms in various complexes, especially those of alkylxanthines (Eckert, 1962; Stamm, 1969; Rohdewald and Baumeister, 1969; Wesselmann, Elmahrouk and Rohdewald, 1982).

From 1935 to 1950 Schüller, together with W. Heubner, was an editor of Heffter's Handbook for experimental Pharmacology.

# *References*

BOEHM, R. (1920). Veratrin und Protoveratrin. In Heffters Handb. exp. Pharmakol., 2, Teil I, 249-282. Berlin: Springer.

CORSTEN, H. (1938). Das Schrifttum der zur Zeit an der Universität Köln wirkenden Dozenten. 136-137. Köln.

ECKERT, Th. (1962). Über Pi-Elektronen-Donor-Acceptor-Komplexe des Procain-Hydrochlorids mit Alkylxanthinen: Untersuchungen zur Frage des Acceptor Zentrums. Arch. Pharm. (Weinheim) 295, 233-240.

FORST, A. W. (1966). Entgiftung. In: Physiologische Chemie (Hrsg. B. Flaschenträger & E. Lehnartz), 2, 2. Teil – Bandteil d/alpha, pp. 1-658 and VIII – XXX. Berlin-Heidelberg-New York: Springer.

HAMACHER, J. (1970). Zur Geschichte der Pharmakologischen Institute der Universität Köln. Das Pharmakologische Institut der Universität Köln – In memoriam Hans Friedrich Zipf. Medizinhistorische Schriftenreihe, 31-34. Mannheim: Boehringer Mannheim.

LABES, R. & RUTENBECK, H. (1933). Die Komplexkonstante der Reaktion zwischen Novokain und Coffein. Arch. exp. Path. Pharmakol., 169, 557-575.

LINDNER, J. (1957). Zeittafeln zur Geschichte der pharmakologischen Institute des deutschen Sprachgebietes. Aulendorf i. Württ.: Editio Cantor.

POGGENDORFF, J. C. (1960). Schüller, Josef. Biogr.-Liter. Hdwrtb., VIIa, 287.

ROHDEWALD, P. & BAUMEISTER, M. (1969). Heats of reaction and stability of caffeine complexes. J. Pharm. Pharmac., 21, 867-869.

SCHÜLLER, J. (1911a). Über Phlorhizin- und Phloretin-Glukuronsäure. 1. Z. Biol., 56, 274-308.

SCHÜLLER, J. (1911b). Automatische Zentren und Reflexvorgänge im abgelösten Darm. Pflügers Arch. ges. Physiol., 141, 133-148.

SCHÜLLER, J, (1921). Über physiologische und pharmakologische Versuche am Rektum des Frosches. Arch. exp. Path. Pharmakol., 90, 196-241.

SCHÜLLER, J. (1922a). Über den Antagonismus der Lokalanästhetika gegenüber dem Veratrineffekt am Muskel. Arch. exp. Path. Pharmakol., 92, XIII.

SCHÜLLER, J. (1922b). Über den Antagonismus einiger Lokalanästhetika gegenüber der Coffeinstarre des Muskels. Arch. exp. Path. Pharmakol., 92, XIII.

SCHÜLLER, J. (1923). Studien über Entgiftungsvorgänge im Organismus. Arch. exp. Path. Pharmakol., 96, II-IV.

SCHÜLLER, J. (1925a). Warum verhindern die Lokalanästhetika die Coffeinstarre des Muskels? Arch. exp. Path. Pharmakol., 105, 224-237.

SCHÜLLER, J. (1925b). Über den Antagonismus einiger Lokalanästhetika gegenüber dem Coffeineffekt am Muskel. Arch. exp. Path. Pharmakol., 105, 299-306.

SCHÜLLER, J. (1925c). Über die Entgiftungspaarungen im Organismus. Arch. exp. Path. Pharmakol., 106, 265-275.

SCHÜLLER, J. (1926). Gift und Gegengift am Muskel. Arch. exp. Path. Pharmakol., 111, 33-34.

SCHÜLLER, J. (1930). Einige Beziehungen zwischen chemischer Konstitution und pharmakologischer Wirkung. Arch. exp. Path. Pharmakol., 147, 64-66.

SCHÜLLER, J. (1935-1950). Mitherausgeber/Coeditor: Heffter's Handb. exp. Pharmakol., Ergänzungswerk, 1-10 (Eds.: W. Heubner & J. Schüller), Berlin: Springer.

SCHÜLLER J. & ATHMER, F. (1921). Über den Antagonismus der Lokalanästhetika gegenüber dem Veratrineffekt am Muskel. Arch. exp. Path. Pharmakol., 91, 125-129.

STAMM, H. (1969). Die kernresonanzspektrographische Untersuchung der Assoziation von Coffein mit Natriumbenzoat und einigen anderen Verbindungen. Arch. Pharm. (Weinheim) 302, 174-184.

WESSELMANN, G., ELMAHROUK, G. & ROHDEWALD, P. (1982). Die dampfdruckosmometrische Bestimmung der Stöchiometrie von Coffein-Komplexen nach der Methode von Asmus. Pharmazie, 37, 639-640.

ZIPF, K. (1930). Über kontrakturerregende Muskelgifte. IV. Die Aufhebung der Coffeinwirkung durch Natriumsalizylat und Natriumbenzoat. Arch. exp. Path. Pharmakol., 149, 94-104.

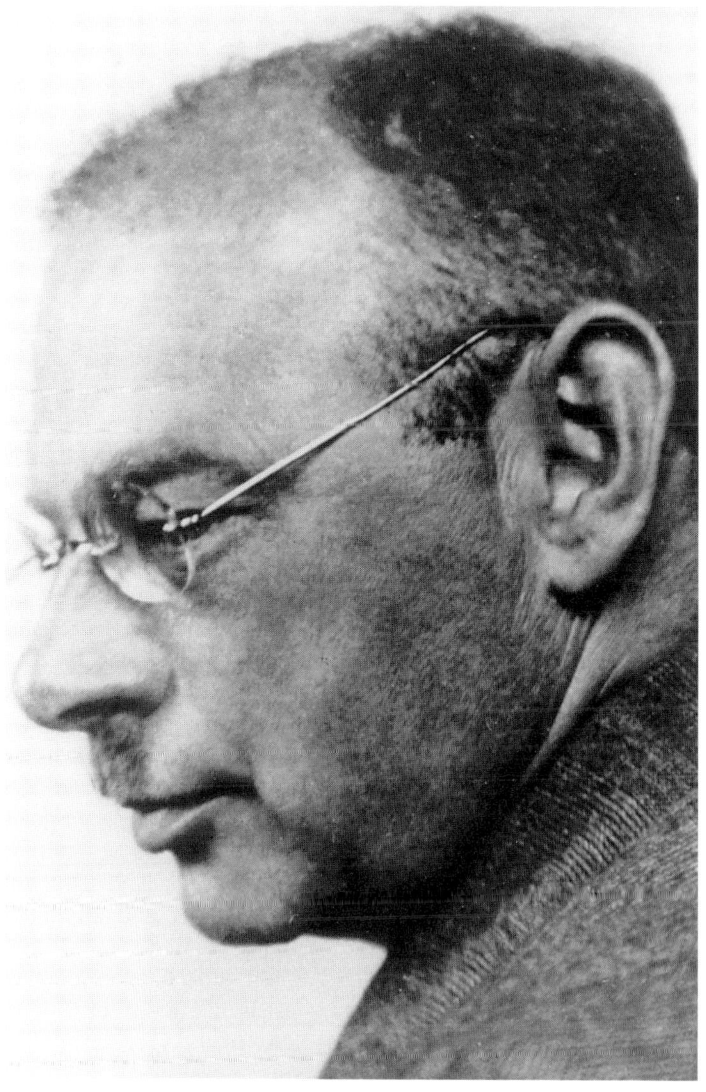

*Fritz Külz*

# Fritz Külz
# 1887 – 1949[*]

Fritz Külz was born on March 7, 1887, in Marburg where his father, Rudolf Eduard Külz was Professor of Physiology. Fritz Külz studied medicine in Freiburg, München, Marburg and Berlin from 1906 to 1912. After having taken his final examination in Marburg, he spent the first part of his internship in the Department of Pathology of that university (under M. B. Schmidt) and the clinical part in a hospital in Bonn. After qualification as a physician (in December 1913) he became Assistant to Max Rubner in the Department of Physiology of the University of Berlin; on July 31, 1914, he was awarded the degree of Dr. med., on the basis of the thesis "On the metabolic energy of some nucleic acids and their degradation products". His further training was interrupted for five years by the First World War and by his contracting lung tuberculosis. During the war he was occupied mainly with investigations of war gases and working in military hospitals.

When Fritz Külz became Assistant to Rudolf Boehm in the Department of Pharmacology of the University of Leipzig in 1919, he was already 32 years old. At the time of his promotion to Lecturer in Pharmacology (November 1922), on the basis of his thesis "Quantitative investigations of the action of homologous quaternary aliphatic ammonium bases" (Külz, 1923), Boehm had already become professor emeritus (1921), and Hermann Fühner had taken over as head of the department (1921–24). Boehm's pupil, Oscar Gros, had taken the chair in Leipzig (1925–1943), and one year later (1926) Fritz Külz went to Kiel as the successor of Oscar Gros as head of the Department of

---

[*]  Biographical sources: Heubner, 1950, Koll et al., 1950; Gelbke, 1956; Lindner, 1957; Poggendorff, 1957; Kroker-Wawrzinek, 1977.

Pharmacology. In 1935 Külz was appointed to the chair at the University of Frankfurt am Main, and he died there on November 2, 1949.

From the very beginning, Fritz Külz's scientific interest was directed towards fundamental, theoretical problems of pharmacology and especially the relationship between chemical structure and biological response. Structure-activity relationships were investigated in various series of inorganic and organic substances from widely different chemical classes. Thanks to his excellent chemical knowledge he was able to synthesize some of these substances himself. Aliphatic quaternary ammonium bases belonged to these series, as did caesium, metal complexes, alkaloids (like papaverine and its derivatives, and apomorphine), and catecholamines.

From these studies of Fritz Külz it emerged that, within homologous series of agents, certain responses change with increasing chain length; responses may increase to a maximum, then decrease with a further increase in chain length or they may be suddenly reversed. As an example one could name the reversal of the vasoconstrictor (or alpha-) effect to a vasodilator (or beta-) effect in the series norepinephrine – epinephrine – isoproterenol. In this context Fritz Külz himself synthesized nylidrine [Dilatol®], a sympathomimetic amine with pronounced vasodilator (or beta-) effects (Külz and Schneider, 1950).


Fritz Külz's studies of homologous series of substances also led him to discover new actions of certain drugs. For instance, tetraethylammonium (TEA) was found to have atropine-like effects on the frog rectum (Schüller, 1921) and on the frog heart (Kulz, 1922), which were interpreted as an antagonistic effect at the muscarinic cholinoceptors. It is of interest to note that Gillespie and Tilmisany (1976) proposed a similar interpretation for the competitive interaction between carbachol and TEA on the anococcygeus muscle of the rat.

# *References*

GELBKE, N. (1956). Die geschichtliche Entwicklung des Pharmakologischen Instituts der Leipziger Universität unter besonderer Berücksichtigung der Gründerjahre. Inaugural-Diss. Leipzig.

GILLESPIE, J. S. & TILMISANY, A. K. (1976). The action of TEA chloride on the response of the rat anococcygeus muscle to motor and inhibitor stimulation and to some drugs. Br. J. Pharmacol., 58, 47-55.

HEUBNER, W. (1950). Eröffnungsansprache. Arch. exp. Path. Pharmakol., 212, 1-8.

KOLL, W., VOGT, W., SCHNEIDER, M. & WIEMERS, K. (1950). In memoriam Fritz Külz. Arch. exp. Path. Pharmakol., 212, 141-144.

KROKER-WAWRZINEK, C. (1977). Die Entwicklung der Pharmakologie und des Pharmakologischen Institutes der Kieler Christiana Albertina (1855-1964). Inaugural-Diss. Kiel.

KÜLZ, F. (1922). Quantitative Untersuchungen über die Wirksamkeit homologer quartärer Ammoniumbasen. Kurze Mitteilung. Pflügers Arch. ges. Physiol., 195, 623-625.

KÜLZ, F. (1923). Quantitative Untersuchungen über die Wirkung homologer quartärer aliphatischer Ammoniumbasen. Arch. exp. Path. Pharmakol., 98, 339-369.

KÜLZ, F. & SCHNEIDER, M. (1950). Neue gefäßerweiternde Sympathicomimetica. Klin. Wschr., 28, 535-537.

LINDNER, J. (1957). Zeittafeln zur Geschichte der pharmakologischen Institute des deutschen Sprachgebietes. Aulendorf i. Württ.: Editio Cantor.

POGGENDORFF, J. C. (1957). Külz, Alexander Rudolf Friedrich Karl (Fritz). Biogr.-Liter. Hdwrtb., VIIa.

SCHÜLLER, J. (1921). Über physiologische und pharmakologische Versuche am Rektum des Frosches. Arch. exp. Path. Pharmakol., 90, 196-241.

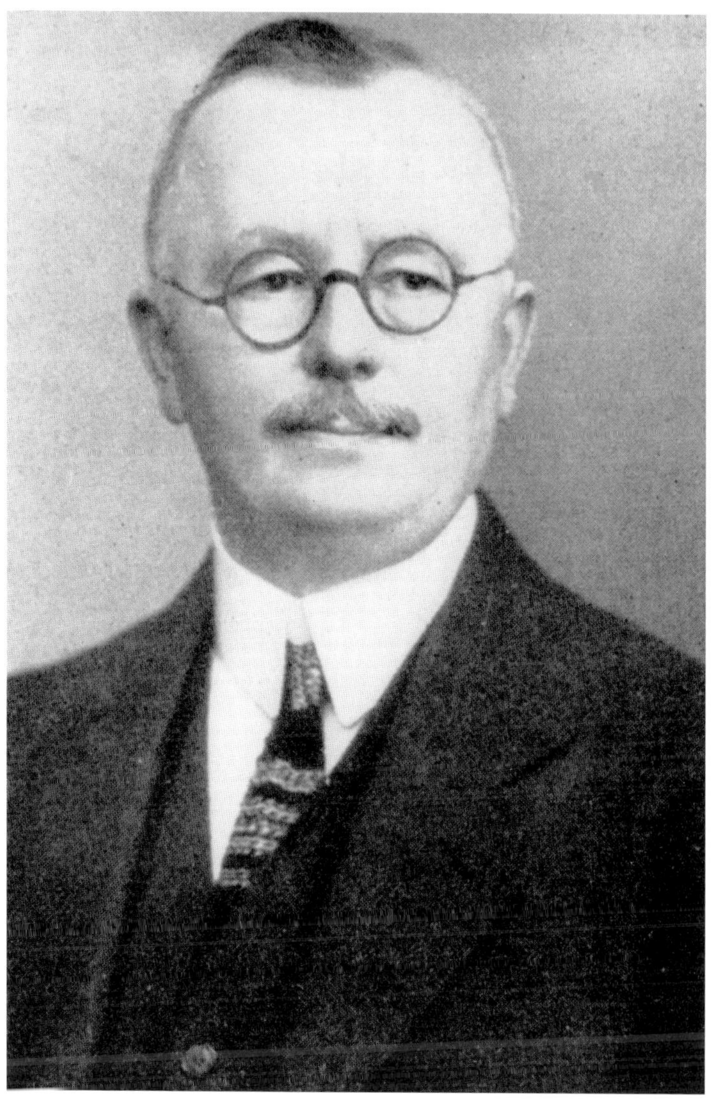

Hermann Fühner

# Hermann Führner
# 1871 – 1944 [*]

Hermann Georg Führner was born at Pforzheim, Baden, on April 10, 1871, the son of a manufacturer of jewelry. In 1887, after six years of high school, he began vocational training in a pharmacy at Kirchheim unter Teck, which he finished in Stuttgart in September 1890 with an examination for 'assistant pharmacists'. Beginning in 1892, he read chemistry at the university of Geneva and received, in the autumn of 1895, the degree of Dr. phil. with the thesis "Recherches sur les indulines et les fluorindines". In 1896 he went to the University of Berlin to study pharmacy and in the spring of 1898 he passed the final high school examination (Abitur), an obligatory prerequisite for the final examination in pharmacy which he passed in the autumn of 1898. Subsequently he read medicine in Berlin; in one year he completed the preclinical course and during the second year he fulfilled his military service obligation by working in the "Hygienisch-chemisches Laboratorium" of the Kaiser-Wilhelm-Akademie. For the remainder of his medical studies he moved to Strassburg where he qualified as a physician in 1902. In the same year he was awarded the degree of Dr. med. with the thesis "Lithotherapie, historische Studien über die medizinische Verwendung der Edelsteine" ["Lithotherapy, historical studies on the medical use of precious stones"] (Führner, 1902). His supervisor was O. Schmiedeberg. The thesis was simultaneously printed in Strassburg and (in an extended version) in Berlin; further editions were published in 1936 and 1956.

---

[*] Biographical references: Führner, 1902; Poggendorff, 1937; Blume, 1941; Hoffmann, 1944; Gelbke, 1956; Lindner, 1957; Zaunick, 1961; Schulemann, 1992; Karzel, 1995.

In subsequent years, Fühner visited various laboratories, including marine-biological stations, to study the potency of anaesthetic agents. Thus, he worked in the Biologische Anstalt on Helgoland in 1903 and 1906, in the Laboratoire Russe de Zoologie in Villefranche sur Mer, France, in 1904, in the Laboratoire Zoologique in Roscoff, Bretagne, in 1905, in the Biologische Versuchsanstalt Prater and the Institute of Pharmacology of the University of Wien in 1906, and finally in the Zoological Station in Napoli in 1908.

Encouraged by Hans Horst Meyer, head of the Department of Pharmacology of the University of Wien since 1904, Fühner began studies on the possible curare-like action of dyes consisting of ammonium bases with a quaternary nitrogen. Such an action was found for methylgreen (Fühner 1906, 1908a), but this substance failed to fulfil the expectation of being able to stain the site of action.

In 1907 Fühner moved to Würzburg as an assistant to Walther Straub, whom he followed to Freiburg i. Br. in 1907; he qualified as Lecturer in Pharmacology in the same year. In 1913 he obtained the title of Professor in Freiburg. During the First World War he served as "Oberapotheker der Reserve" but this did not prevent him from being asked to take over the Department of Pharmacology of the University of Königsberg in 1915. In 1921 he was appointed to the chair in Leipzig as the successor of the retired mentor of pharmacology, Rudolf Boehm. Thus, Fühner directed one of the largest and best equipped pharmacological departments in Germany. However, he did not stay long in Leipzig, since he moved to the University of Bonn in 1924. He retired at the end of 1936, but remained director until the autumn of 1937. He died in Bonn on January 11, 1944.

As a Privatdozent (Lecturer) in Freiburg Fühner gave demonstration lectures in pharmacology for chemists and pharmacists. During their studies, his students became acquainted with chemical methods for the detection of certain poisons, and it was his aim to convince them of the efficiency of biological-pharmacological approaches. He realized that the number of biological detection methods was relatively small and he embarked on the development of new methods for the detection and the quantitative measurement of agents of pharmacological and toxicological/forensic importance. The external conditions were favourable, since his teacher Straub was convinced of the need for the development and use of isolated organ preparations as tools for the quantitative evaluation of substances based on their biological responses. Moreover, Straub was busy planning the new Freiburg department as a modern and spacious research institute, which included an efficient mechanical workshop devoted to the development of apparatus.

Fühner soon recognized the lack of any compendium of the then available biological methods used for the identification and the quantitative measurement of poisons. He decided to publish a review of the qualitative assays of poisons as well as of the quantitative methods used for the measurements of drugs. This led to the monograph "Nachweis und Bestimmung von Giften auf biologischem Wege, eine Anleitung für Pharmakologen, Gerichtsärzte, Gerichtschemiker und Apotheker" ["Detection and characterization of poisons by biological methods; a guide for pharmacologists, forensic physicians, forensic chemists and pharmacists"] (Fühner, 1911a). In his preface Fühner expresses his gratitude to the head of the department, W. Straub, for the financial support provided by the department during the preliminary work, and to his colleague P. Trendelenburg for his kind help. Paul Trendelenburg had worked for his Dr. med. under Straub (1908) and had been in the department as an Assistant since 1909. His method for the quantitative measurement of adrenaline in blood (Trendelenburg, 1910) appears in the monograph as well as the biological assay methods, developed by Fühner himself, for guanidine (Fühner, 1907), colchicine (Fühner, 1910) and aconitine (Fühner, 1911b); he also reported the leech preparation (Fühner, 1909), first developed because of its high sensitivity to nicotine which would later turn out to be of special importance (see below). Finally, his monograph contained the quantitative method for the estimation of synthetic muscarine on the isolated toad heart, developed at the Zoological Station in Napoli (Fühner, 1908b).

While investigating the effects of extracts of the posterior pituitary lobe in whole animals, Fühner (1913) observed the simultaneous appearance of an apnoea and a rise in blood pressure; similar effects were elicited by adrenaline, administered for comparison. These observations led him to study the effects of adrenaline on the pulmonary circulation in the heart-lung preparation which permitted control of the arterial resistance and venous return as well as the continuous recording of stroke volume and peripheral and pulmonary arterial pressure. Fühner managed to interest E. H. Starling in this project and, in the Department of Physiology at University College, London, the two of them carried out experiments on the heart-lung preparation as well as on the isolated, perfused lung (Fühner and Starling, 1913). They defined the relationship between pulmonary and systemic arterial pressure and the effects of asphyxia and carbon dioxide on arterial pressure in parallel to the function of the heart, as well as the pressor effect of adrenaline in the pulmonary artery as a consequence of the constriction of pulmonary blood vessels.

In the further pursuit of the development of biological assay methods, Fühner whilst in Königsberg concentrated on acetylcholine. In order to assay small amounts of choline in animal tissues, Guggenheim and Löffler (1916) had converted this compound of relatively low potency into the very potent acetylcholine; the latter was then assayed on the isolated ileum of the guinea pig. Fühner preferred for his assay the isolated heart of the frog which is not only more sensitive to acetylcholine than the guinea-pig ileum, but permits a greater number of exposures

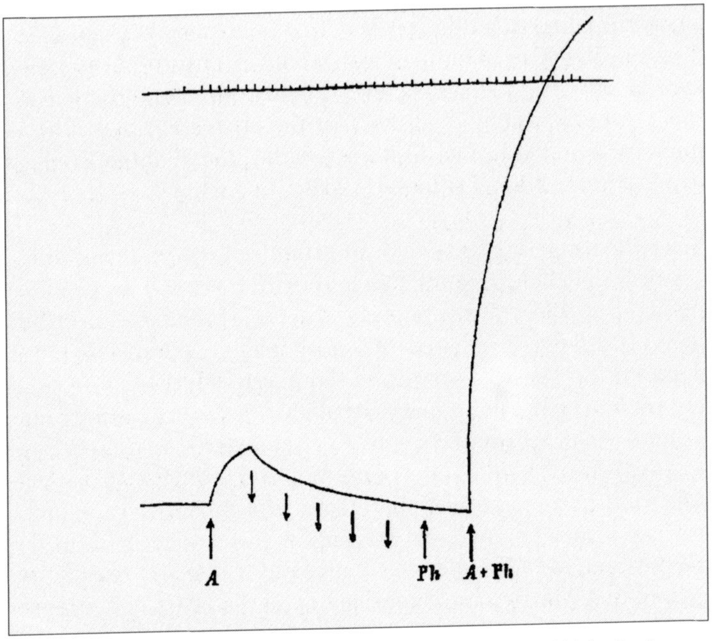



*Tracing of leech smooth muscle. A – acetylcholine 1 : 1,000,000 for 5 min. Downward arrow – wash-out. Ph – physostigmine 1 : 1,000,000 for 5 min. A + Ph – mixture of both. Time in min. From Fühner, 1917b.*

to drugs. Thus, with the frog heart it is possible to calibrate the preparation before a solution with unknown concentration is assayed (Fühner, 1916). On this preparation acetylcholine turned out to be about 100,000 times more potent than choline. Probably because of the ongoing war, Fühner realized only later that Reid Hunt had already used the isolated heart of the frog to assay choline, following its conversion to acetylcholine (Hunt, 1915).

In a series of publications "Investigations of the synergism of poisons" he tested the ability of various substances with respect to their response-enhancing effects on smooth muscle (Fühner,

1917a). He found that acetylcholine, in contrast to its effect on the isolated heart of the frog, was only weakly effective on the isolated leech muscle. "The weak stimulatory effect of acetylcholine, which appears to be reduced to the level of that of choline, can be enhanced one million-fold by physostigmine in concentrations which are solely response-enhancing [but not active on their own], while the effect of choline is not enhanced." This potentiation of the effects of the choline ester is "the strongest yet known true synergism" (Fühner, 1922). Fühner had a clear picture of the mechanism of action of physostigmine: "This extraordinary potentiation appears to have a simple chemical explanation", provided one considers "that acetylcholine, which is unstable especially in alkaline solution, is split into choline and acetic acid at its site of action; the degradation is prevented by physostigmine. This is indicated by experiments with acids which also enhanced the effect of acetylcholine" (Fühner, 1917a).

With his discovery of the extraordinary potentiation of the effects of acetylcholine, resulting from the inhibition of its hydrolysis by physostigmine (see Figure from Fühner, 1917b), Fühner without doubt created the methodological basis for the clarification of the role of acetylcholine as a transmitter of neuronal impulses, which was confirmed by a series of publications in rapid succession (Loewi and Navratil, 1926; Feldberg, 1933; Feldberg and Krayer, 1933; Krayer and Verney, 1934, 1935; Feldberg and Gaddum, 1934; Dale and Feldberg, 1934). In all these studies the researchers measured either the sensitization by physostigmine of physiological responses to nerve stimulation or the contraction of the leech muscle sensitized by physostigmine. In the absence of any chemical method for the identification of acetylcholine, positive results were first interpreted in terms of evidence for an "acetylcholine-like" substance. This changed after Dale (1935) pointed out that, even in the absence of a chemical method, the identification of the substance can be achieved by physiological methods with a high degree of probability. "Taken together, the evidence is now very strong that the peripheral transmitter involved in responses to parasympathetic nerve stimulation is indeed acetylcholine, and it does not seem to be any longer necessary to speak of an acetylcholine-like substance" (Dale, 1935). For the demonstration of the humoral transmission of nerve impulses Sir Henry Dale and Otto Loewi received the Nobel Prize in 1936. In his publications, Dale himself referred to the fundamental importance of Fühner's discovery of the potentiation of the effects of acetylcholine by physostigmine and of the inhibition of the hydrolytic degradation of acetylcholine by this substance (Dale and Gaddum, 1930; Dale, 1935).

Fühner's experiments with barium chloride (Fühner, 1917a, 1917c) yielded results which, in the context of the effect of physostigmine, first appeared uninterpretable; however, with today's knowledge of the role of acetylcholine as a transmitter an interpretation is now possible. Fühner had found that barium chloride ("baryt") contracted the smooth muscle of the leech which, though free of ganglion cells, still contained nerve endings (Fühner, 1917c). On frog skeletal muscle this contractile effect was not obtained after degeneration of the motor nerves, although the muscle still retained its responsiveness to acetylcholine (Fühner, 1917c, 1920a). The response of the leech muscle to barium chloride was potentiated by physostigmine to the same extent as that to acetylcholine (Fühner, 1917a, 1917c). Since "an identical site of action on the leech muscle is unlikely for acetylcholine and baryt" (Fühner, 1917a), and since degeneration of the motor nerves prevented any effect of barium, one can conclude that barium acts on motor nerve endings to release acetylcholine, the effect of which on the leech muscle is then potentiated by physostigmine. Thus, physostigmine revealed the transmitter acetylcholine in situ. Fühner later extended his studies into the effects of barium on motor nerve endings (Fühner, 1927) and found that they were antagonized by calcium and magnesium chloride, similarly to guanidine's ability to elicit muscle twitches by acting on nerve endings (Fühner, 1907, 1925a).

A central theme in Fühner's research was the question of the relationship between the anaesthetic effect of substances and their molecular properties. He studied the inhibition by alcohols of the development of fertilized eggs of the sea urchin (Fühner, 1903, 1904). In agreement with Overton's observations on tadpoles (1901), he found a "pharmacological rule", according to which the effectiveness among a homologous series of monovalent, saturated primary alcohols increases from ethyl to heptyl alcohol; moreover, when expressed in molar amounts, each member of this series appears to be 3 times more potent than the preceding one (Fühner, 1904). He found the same relationship in studies of the haemolysis of bovine erythrocytes (Fühner and Neubauer, 1907). Tests on various marine animals later showed that the potency ratio was not always exactly 3, but varied between 3 and 4, with a mean of 3.6 (Fühner, 1912).

Already in 1904 J. Traube had pointed out that the rule observed by Fühner in animal experiments corresponded to a physicochemical rule described by himself. He wrote: "Similar equivalents of substances of homologous series with capillary activity (common alcohols, fatty acids, esters) reduce the height of the water column [in a capillary tube] in the proportion $1 : 3 : 3^2 : 3^3 ...$" (Traube, 1904). This prompted him to regard the surface activity of a substance as the determinant of its anaesthetising activity, in constrast to Hans H. Meyer's (1899) and Overton's (1901) postulated relation to lipid solubility. Fühner later studied the anaesthetic effect of "light benzines", i.e., the carbohydrates pentane, hexane, heptane and octane (Fühner, 1921a); he found that their anaesthetic activity in white mice also increased by a factor of 3, with simultaneous decrease of their water solubility in the proportion $1 : 3 : 3^2$, but without any change in their surface activity. Hence, Fühner's rule of activity in homologous series proved to be independent of Traube's rule of capillary activity.

Complementary studies of anaesthetic activity, surface tension and water solubility of halogen-free and halogen-containing substances acting on the isolated heart of the frog (Fühner, 1921b) as well as studies of their haemolytic activity (Fühner, 1923a) confirmed the parallelism between pharmacological effect and water solubility; in contrast, determinations of the surface tension according to Traube revealed no proportionality to the anaesthetic activity, except for alcohols and related substances. Hence, in homologous series water solubility apparently declines by a constant factor and this general rule appears to be of greater biological importance than Traube's rule concerning capillary activity. From these experiments the general conclusion was reached that "molar water solubility declined in homologous series of organic compounds in such a way that each member was 3–4 times less water soluble [and correspondingly more lipid soluble] than the preceding one" (Fühner, 1924a).

While he was head of the department in Leipzig, Fühner's monograph of 1911 appeared as a contribution to the Handbuch der biologischen Arbeitsmethoden, ed. by Abderhalden, under the more explicit title "Detection and measurement of poisons by pharmacological methods"(Fühner, 1923b). This article was supplemented by methods for the quantitative estimation of acetylcholine and choline (Fühner, 1916) as well as for the identification of physostigmine and nicotine on the leech muscle (Fühner, 1918a,b). Later, there followed a report on the assay of cathartics in white mice (Fühner, 1925b). He contributed reviews dealing with colchicine (Fühner, 1920b), muscarines, guanidines and organic dyes (Fühner, 1923c,d,e) to Heffter's Handbuch der experimentellen Pharmakologie.

In October 1924 Fühner became director of the Department of Pharmacology in Bonn, which was unsatisfactorily housed in a building which, until 1890, had served pathology. In a contribution "Das pharmakologische Institut" to the History of the University of Bonn, Fühner offered a valuable review of the development of pharmacology in German universities in the 19th century as well as a vivid description of his new abode: "The best part of the building still is its basement with its large, vaulted rooms with high ceilings, the constant temperature of which is not only optimally suited for keeping the large number of frogs, housed in several containers with constant flow of water, but, in the past, also to the innkeepers of the neighbourhood for storing their wine. In pre-war times clever "Institutsdiener" are said to have grown cultures of mushrooms which acquired widespread fame because of their excellence." He ended with the statement: "Only a new building, planned since 1924, will ensure that pharmacology can be taught in Bonn with modern equipment and be advanced scientifically" (Fühner, 1933).

These conditions probably contributed to Fühner's pronounced literary activity in Bonn, to which belongs a historical-ethnological study "Solanaceae as intoxicants" (Fühner, 1926). This was initiated by a case of intoxication with Scopolia carniolica in Lithuania, on which he was asked to provide an expert opinion. His colleague in Heidelberg, Hermann Wieland, who unfortunately died early, "had the idea to collect cases of intoxications and to publish them in a suitable form". Fühner followed up this suggestion by publishing the "Sammlung von Vergiftungsfällen" (Fühner, 1930) with the support of the German Pharmacological Society as well as of the pharmacologists Erich Hesse in Breslau and Emil Starkenstein in Prag. The first volume of this journal (with 12 issues) appeared in 1930. Fühner asked Wieland's pupil, the pharmacologist Behrend Behrens in Kiel, to become editor in 1935. From 1936, the year of Fühner's retirement, this journal carried the title "Fühner-Wielands Sammlung von Vergiftungs-fällen", from volume 15 it has been titled "Archiv für Toxikologie".

When, in 1924, a lecture in pharmacology was incorporated into the curriculum for pharmacy students, Fühner, at that time in Leipzig, had pleaded that all departments of pharmacology offer one lecture per week to pharmacists. Moreover, following the example of his predecessor Boehm, he argued for tying pharmacognosy to pharmacology. He proposed that pharmacognosy units be established in university departments of pharmacology in which a pharmacist with chemistry and botany training would be responsible for the teaching of the subject, while at the same time carrying out pharmacognosy research in collaboration with the pharmacologist, i.e., searching for the active substances in medicinal plants. "Pharmacognosy must no longer be surrendered to the botanists under whose guidance it will stultify in methodological minutiae." This association with pharmacology "should last until independent departments of pharmacognosy can be built in all universities" (Fühner, 1924b).

From the end of 1934 pharmacy students had to pass an examination in pharmacology. Fühner therefore decided to write a textbook "Pharmakologie für Pharmazeuten", in which drugs are not grouped according to their chemical classes, as pharmacists are used to, but according to their medical use, i.e., to their indications; this will be more helpful for pharmacists, who wish to acquaint themselves with their effects (Fühner, 1937). Further editions of this book were published in 1940 and 1948.

After this textbook for pharmacists, Fühner, now retired, wrote "Medizinische Toxikologie" as a "textbook for physicians, pharmacists and chemists" (Fühner, 1943). This book with 250 pages was published in the year before his death. A renowned contemporary toxicologist wrote: " This 'Toxikologie' has been written with such judgement, precision, reliability and with such brevity, as it is possible only for an author who spent his whole academic life with this topic. Fühner has developed and extended methods for the identification of poisons by pharmacological experiments, has a thorough knowledge of the relevant literature through the 'Sammlung von Vergiftungsfällen' founded by him and has sharpened his judgement by providing many expert opinions for law suits; in short, he has an overview over the whole field and he may well regard the material presented here as his most beloved brainchild arising from his research and his lectures" (Rost, 1943). The second edition, revised by Fühner, appeared in 1947, a third edition in 1951 was edited by Wolfgang Wirth and Gerhard Hecht. In 1967 the book appeard in a new form and under the title "Toxikologie-Fibel" with the three authors W. Wirth, G. Hecht and Chr. Gloxhuber.

Fühner was convinced that a large number of physicians was ignorant of the symptomatology of intoxication as a prerequisite for their diagnosis and that an improvement of toxicological teaching was indispensable. He regarded as essential special toxicology lectures, presented by pharmacologists, in which the physician would not only learn the diverse possibilities of intoxication and to differentiate the symptom complexes, but be instructed in the symptomatic and causal therapy of intoxications (Fühner, 1943).


## *References*

BLUME, W. (1941). Hermann Fühner zum siebzigsten Geburtstag. Klin. Wschr., Berlin, 20, 351-352.

DALE, Sir H. (1935). Reizübertragung durch chemische Mittel im peripheren Nervensystem. Sammlung d. Nothnagel-Vorträge, Heft 4, 1-23. Berlin / Wien: Urban & Schwarzenberg.

DALE, H. H. & FELDBERG, W. (1934). The chemical transmitter of vagus effects to the stomach. J. Physiology, 81, 320-334.

DALE, H. H. & GADDUM, J. H. (1930). Reactions of denervated voluntary muscle, and their bearing on the mode of action of parasympathetic and related nerves. J. Physiology, 70, 109-144.

FELDBERG, W. (1933). Der Nachweis eines acetylcholinähnlichen Stoffes im Zungenvenenblut des Hundes bei Reizung des Nervus lingualis. Pflugers Arch. ges. Physiol., 232, 88-104.

FELDBERG, W. & GADDUM, J. H. (1934). The chemical transmitter at synapses in a sympathetic ganglion. J. Physiology, 81, 305-319.

FELDBERG, W. & KRAYER, O. (1933). Das Auftreten eines azetylcholinartigen Stoffes im Herzvenenblut von Warmblütern bei Reizung der Nervi vagi. Arch. exp. Path. Pharmakol., 172, 170-193.

FÜHNER, H. (1902). Lithotherapie. Historische Studien über die medizinische Verwendung der Edelsteine. 118+1 pp., Inaugural-Diss., Strassburg i. E.

FÜHNER, H. (1903). Über die Einwirkung verschiedener Alkohole auf die Entwicklung der Seeigel. Arch. exp. Path. Pharmakol., 51, 1-10.

FÜHNER, H. (1904). Pharmakologische Studien an Seeigeleiern. Der Wirkungsgrad der Alkohole. Arch. exp. Path. Pharmakol., 52, 69-82.

FÜHNER, H. (1906). Ein physiologischer Beitrag zur Frage der Constitution der Farbammoniumbasen. Ber. Dtsch. chem. Ges., 39, 2437-2438.

FÜHNER, H. (1907). Curarestudien, 1. Die periphere Wirkung des Guanidins. Arch. exp. Path. Pharmakol., 58, 1-49.

FÜHNER, H. (1908a). Curarestudien, 2. Die Wirkung des Methylgrüns. Arch. exp. Path. Pharmakol., 59, 161-178.

FÜHNER, H. (1908b). Die quantitative Bestimmung des synthetischen Muskarins auf physiologischem Wege. Arch. exp. Path. Pharmakol., 59, 179-185.

FÜHNER, H. (1909). Über den Antagonismus Nikotin-Curare. Pflügers Arch. ges. Physiol., 129, 107-109.

FÜHNER, H. (1910). Über den toxikologischen Nachweis des Colchicins. Arch. exp. Path. Pharmakol., 63, 357-373.

FÜHNER, H. (1911a). Nachweis und Bestimmung von Giften auf biologischem Wege. 176 pp., Berlin / Wien: Urban & Schwarzenberg.

FÜHNER, H. (1911b). Über den toxikologischen Nachweis des Aconitins. Arch. exp. Path. Pharmakol., 66, 179-190.

FÜHNER, H. (1912). Der Wirkungsgrad der einwertigen Alkohole. Z. Biologie, 57, 469-494.

FÜHNER, H. (1913). Pharmakologische Untersuchungen über die wirksamen Bestandteile der Hypophyse. Z. ges. exp. Med., 1, 379-443.

FÜHNER, H. (1916). Die quantitative Bestimmung des Cholins auf biologischem Wege. Biochem. Z., 77, 408-414.

FÜHNER, H. (1917a). Untersuchungen über den Synergismus von Giften, 4. Die chemische Erregbarkeitssteigerung glatter Muskulatur. Arch. exp. Path. Pharmakol., 82, 51-80.

FÜHNER, H. (1917b). Ein Vorlesungsversuch zur Demonstration der erregbarkeitssteigernden Wirkung des Physostigmins. Arch. exp. Path. Pharmakol., 82, 81-85.

FÜHNER, H. (1917c). Untersuchungen über die periphere Wirkung des Physostigmins. Arch. exp. Path. Pharmakol., 82, 205-220.

FÜHNER, H. (1918a). Der toxikologische Nachweis des Physostigmins. Biochem. Z., 92, 347-354.

FÜHNER, H. (1918b). Die quantitative Bestimmung des Nicotins auf biologischem Wege. Biochem. Z., 92, 355-363.

FÜHNER, H. (1920a). Untersuchungen über den Synergismus von Giften, 5. Guanidin-Barytmischungen. Arch. exp. Path. Pharmakol., 88, 179-191.

FÜHNER, H. (1920b). Die Colchicingruppe. Handb. exp. Pharmakol. (Heffter), 2, 1, 493-507.

FÜHNER, H. (1921a). Die narkotische Wirkung des Benzins und seiner Bestandteile (Pentan, Hexan, Heptan, Octan). Biochem. Z., 115, 235-261.

FÜHNER, H. (1921b). Die Wirkungsstärke der Narkotica, 1. Versuche am isolierten Froschherzen. Biochem. Z., 120, 143-163.

FÜHNER, H. (1922). Chemischer und pharmakologischer Synergismus. München. med. Wschr., 69, 915-917.

FÜHNER, H. (1923a). Die Wirkungsstärke der Narkotica, 2. Hämolyseversuche. Biochem. Z., 139, 216-224.

FÜHNER, H. (1923b). Nachweis und Bestimmung von Giften auf pharmakologischem Wege. Handb. biol. Arb.-Meth. (Abderhalden), IV, 7, 1, 461-612.

FÜHNER, H. (1923c). Die Muscaringruppe. Handb. exp. Pharmakol. (Heffter), I., 640-683.

FÜHNER, H. (1923d). Die Guanidingruppe. Handb. exp. Pharmakol. (Heffter), I., 684-701.

FÜHNER, H. (1923e). Die Gruppe der organischen Farbstoffe. Handb. exp. Pharmakol. (Heffter), I., 1199-1296.

FÜHNER, H. (1924a). Die Wasserlöslichkeit in homologen Reihen. Ber. Dtsch. chem. Ges., 57, 510-515.

FÜHNER, H. (1924b). Pharmakologie und Pharmakognosie. Pharm. Ztg., 69, 893.

FÜHNER, H. (1925a). Über die Guanidinkontraktur des Skelettmuskels. Arch. exp. Path. Pharmakol., 105, 265-277.

FÜHNER, H. (1925b). Die pharmakologische Wertbestimmung der Abführmittel. Arch. exp. Path. Pharmakol., 105, 249-263.

FÜHNER, H. (1926). Solanazeen als Berauschungsmittel. Arch. exp. Path. Pharmakol., 111, 281-294.

FÜHNER, H. (1927). Über die Wirkung des Bariumchlorids am Skelettmuskel. Arch. exp. Path. Pharmakol., 119, 56-65.

FÜHNER, H. (1930-1934). Hrsg. Sammlung von Vergiftungsfällen, 1-5, Leipzig.

FÜHNER, H. (1933). Das Pharmakologische Institut. Geschichte der Rheinischen Friedrich-Wilhelm-Universität zu Bonn am Rhein, 2., Institute und Seminare 1818-1933. 83-88. Bonn: Cohen.

FÜHNER, H. (1937). Pharmakologie für Pharmazeuten, 8+235 pp., Berlin; 2 (Berlin 1940); 3(Bln-Frkf/M. 1948) 204 pp., bearb. von R. Hanslian.

FÜHNER, H. (1943). Medizinische Toxikologie, Lehrbuch für Ärzte, Apotheker und Chemiker. 12+295 pp., Leipzig; 2(1947); 3 (Stuttg. 1951) 12+251 pp., bearb. von W. Wirth & G. Hecht.

FÜHNER, H. & NEUBAUER, E. (1907). Hämolyse durch Substanzen homologer Reihen. Arch. exp. Path. Pharmakol., 56, 333-345.

FÜHNER, H. & STARLING, E. H. (1913). Experiments on the pulmonary circulation. J. Physiology, 47, 286-304.

GELBKE, N. (1956). Die geschichtliche Entwicklung des Pharmakologischen Instituts der Leipziger Universität unter besonderer Berücksichtigung der Gründerjahre. Inaugural-Diss., Leipzig.

GUGGENHEIM, M. & LÖFFLER, W. (1916) Eine Methode zum Nachweis kleiner Cholinmengen. Biochem. Z., 74, 208-218.

HOFFMANN, E. (1944). Über den Synergismus von Arzneimitteln. Zum Andenken an H. Fühner. München. med. Wschr., 91, 85-86.

HUNT, R. (1915). A physiological test for cholin and some of its applications. J. Pharmacol, exp. Ther. 7, 301-337.

KARZEL, K. (1995). Geschichte der Pharmakologie und Toxikologie an der Universität Bonn. In Bonner Univ. Bl., Ges. Freunde u. Förd. Univ. Bonn. 69-80.

KRAYER, O. & VERNEY, E. B. (1934). Veränderung des Acetylcholingehaltes im Blute der Coronarvenen unter dem Einfluß einer Blutdrucksteigerung durch Adrenalin. Klin. Wschr., Berlin, 13, 1250-1251.

KRAYER, O. & VERNEY, E. B. (1935). Reflektorische Beeinflussung des Gehaltes an Acetylcholin im Blute der Coronarvenen. Arch. exp. Path. Pharmakol., 180, 75-92.

LINDNER, J. (1957). Zeittafeln zur Geschichte der pharmakologischen Institute des deutschen Sprachgebietes. 167 pp., Aulendorf i. Württ.: Editio Cantor.

LOEWI, O. & NAVRATIL, E. (1926). Über den Mechanismus der Vaguswirkung von Physostigmin und Ergotamin. Pflügers Arch. ges. Physiol., 214, 689-696.

MEYER, H. (1899). Welche Eigenschaft der Anästhetica bedingt ihre narkotische Wirkung? Arch. exp. Path. Pharmakol., 42, 109-118.

OVERTON, E. (1901). Studien über die Narkose. Jena.

POGGENDORFF, J. C. (1937). Fühner, Hermann Georg. Biogr.-Liter. Hdwrtb., VI; (1958) VII a.

ROST, E. (1943). H. FÜHNER, Bonn: Med. Toxikologie. Ein Lehrbuch für Ärzte, Apotheker und Chemiker. Ref. in Dtsch. med. Wschr., 69, 611.

SCHULEMANN, W. (1992). Hermann Fühner, 1871-1944. In Bonner Gelehrte. Beiträge zur Geschichte der Wissenschaften in Bonn; Medizin., 163-167. Bonn.

TRAUBE, J. (1904). Theorie der Osmose und Narkose. Pflügers Arch. ges. Physiol., 105, 541-558.

TRENDELENBURG, P. (1910). Bestimmung des Adrenalingehaltes im normalen Blut sowie beim Abklingen der Wirkung einer einmaligen intravenösen Adrenalininjektion mittels physiologischer Meßmethode. Arch. exp. Path. Pharmakol., 63, 161-176.

ZAUNICK, R. (1961). Fühner, Hermann Georg, Neue Dtsch. Biogr., 5, 687, 120, 143-163.

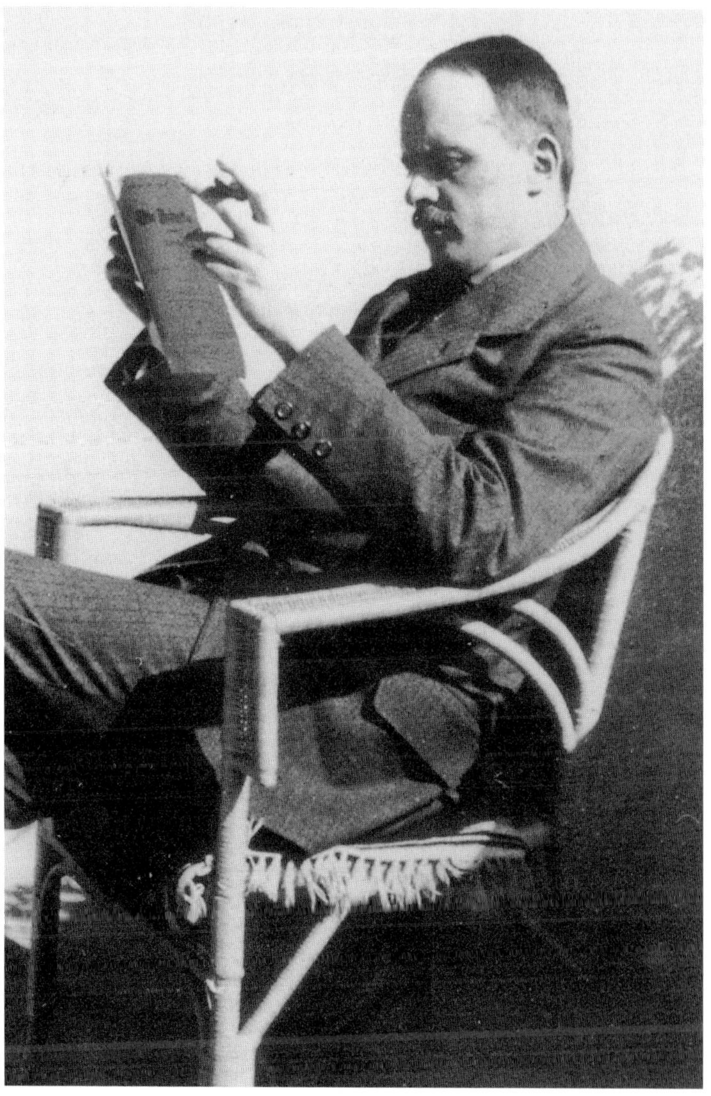

*Paul Trendelenburg*

# Paul Trendelenburg
## 1884 – 1931[*]

Paul Trendelenburg was born at Bonn on March 24, 1884. His father was the famous German surgeon Friedrich Trendelenburg. He began his medical study at Leipzig University in 1903 and completed it in 1907 at the University of Freiburg i. Br. In 1908, as an intern, he spent the first three months in the laboratory of Walther Straub who had been Professor of Pharmacology at Freiburg University since 1907. There he did experimental work on a problem of the pharmacology of digitalis to fulfill some of the requirements for receiving the degree of Dr. of Medicine. In the work for his dissertation "On the mechanism of action and intensity of effect of various cardiac glycosides" Trendelenburg utilized the isolated frog heart described by Straub and studied various cardiac glycosides to compare quantitatively the concentrations leading to the systolic standstill and the time required at varying concentrations to achieve it (Trendelenburg, 1909). As stated above (see chapter on Straub) one of the important results of this study was the discovery that, while increasing concentrations lead to speeding up the occurrence of the endeffect, the time to systolic standstill could not be reduced beyond a definite period. Trendelenburg concluded that the mechanism of the cardiac glycoside effect is biphasic: the physiological final effect which can be recorded is preceded by a physiologically latent chemical action.

For the completion of the medical part of his internship Trendelenburg went to the German Hospital in London. The experimental and clinical experience of his internship year made Tren-

---

[*] Biographical sources: Heubner, 1931; Janssen and Pietrkowski, 1931; Krayer, 1931; Straub, 1931; Stroomann, 1931; Loewi, 1932; Lindner, 1957.

delenburg to choose pharmacology as a career. He returned to Straub at Freiburg in 1909 to become Assistant in Pharmacology and remained in this position until 1919. In 1912 he qualified as Lecturer in Pharmacology and, in 1916, he received the title of Professor. Towards the end of the First World War, from September 15 to November 17, 1918, Trendelenburg was called to the German occupation University of Dorpat (in Estonia) as Professor of Pharmacology but had to relinquish this position after a few months and returned to Freiburg, when the Russians occupied the Baltic States. Shortly after this, Trendelenburg was asked to take over the Department of Pharmacology at Rostock where he stayed from 1919 until 1923. He was the successor of W. Straub as Professor of Pharmacology at Freiburg University from 1923 to 1927. In the summer of 1927 he moved to the University of Berlin to succeed A. Heffter and was head of the Department of Pharmacology until 1930 when he fell ill and he died on February 4, 1931 not yet 47 years of age.

At Freiburg University, as an Assistant to Straub from 1909 to 1919, Paul Trendelenburg became a leading participant in the development and use of isolated organs as pharmacological tools for the purpose of quantitatively measuring drug effects. Of the experimental work he carried out during this time three areas stand out. Firstly, the isolated perfused hindlegs of the frog which had been previously employed by Fraser (1892) to examine whether strophanthus extracts had vasoconstrictive activity. Later Straub suggested to Laewen (1904) to utilize it for the demonstration of the vasoconstrictor action of epinephrine. Then Trendelenburg (1910) developed the preparation for the quantitative determination of epinephrine in body fluids, e.g. blood. Secondly, Trendelenburg (1912) carried out the first systematic pharmacological study of the isolated circular bronchial muscle, which he obtained from the lung of the cow. And thirdly, the small intestine of which Magnus (1904) had used isolated pieces to study the effect of drugs on the pendular movements. Trendelenburg, by using the isolated small intestine of the guinea pig, arranged the preparation so that it became possible to alter and measure intraluminal pressure. He discovered the initiation of peristaltic movements by increasing intraluminal pressure. His systematic studies of this preparation led to the famous publication entitled "Physiologische und pharmakologische Versuche über die Dünndarmperistaltik" (Trendelenburg, 1917).

For the development of Trendelenburg's work as a whole, the frog hindleg preparation was of particular importance. In a series of about 20 publications he examined the epinephrine content of the blood, presumably resulting from the internal secretion of the suprarenal medulla, under various physiological, pathological and pharmacological conditions. This was Paul Trendelenburg's first step into the field of internal secretion in general. Moreover, the occupation with epinephrine and its powerful circulatory effects, as his earlier occupation with cardioactive substances of the digitalis series, introduced him to the problems of the physiology and pharmacology of the circulation that provided many challenges for his superb experimental skills. In the Rostock period (1919–23), the studies on catecholamine secretion were continued. In comprehensive surveys of the literature and of his own work Trendelenburg (1923, 1924) reviewed his extensive experience with, and knowledge of, the function of the suprarenal medulla under normal and altered conditions. His interest also turned to two new fields of exploration: the pituitary body and the function of the parathyroids.

Using the isolated uterus of various laboratory animals (e. g., guinea pig, rat) the evaluation of the oxytocic principle of the posterior lobe was given special attention. A therapeutically useful result of the development of the quantitative methods of assay was the recognition of extreme variability and even complete inactivity of drugs distributed by the pharmaceutical industry for their oxytocic activity (Trendelenburg, 1922). His work called for standardization of oxytocic activity and terminated the sale of inactive preparations in Germany.

The problem of tetany after thyroidectomy was examined by following the $Ca^{2+}$ concentration in the blood serum of experimental animals. For the quantitative determination of the change in Ca ion concentration a bioassay using the isolated frog heart was employed after its suitability for this purpose had been established by examining its sensitivity and accuracy (Trendelenburg and Goebel, 1921).

It was during this time that Trendelenburg conceived the plan to review the physiology and pharmacology of the hormones in an attempt to sift facts from conjecture and fantasy in this field. His aim was to continue his own studies and to try basing his conclusions upon proven facts and quantitative data of his own laboratory as well as on those of the literature. In the Freiburg period (1923–27), Trendelenburg's prodigious literary work on the hormone book started in earnest. To a large extent the experimental work of the laboratory also dealt with endocrinological problems. The problem of supersensitivity to epinephrine was examined after acute and chronic denervation of sympathetically innervated effector organs (Shimidzu, 1924). Tetany after the selective removal of the parathyroids was further examined and the change in Ca ion concentration in blood followed also by chemical determination (Schulten, 1925a,b). At this time parathormone, a potent parathyroid preparation (Collip, 1925), became available and was used to examine its effects on bone metabolism (Bülbring, 1931). Distribution and elimination of iodine after parenteral administration of thyroglobulin and thyroxine was followed in rats. A considerable part was excreted in the bile still in organic combination so as to cause metamorphosis in the axolotl (Krayer, 1928). The function of skeletal muscle was examined after extirpation of the suprarenal cortex and the remedial effect of cortex extracts studied (Kühl, 1927).

Most attention was given by Trendelenburg and several of his coworkers during this period to the function of the posterior lobe of the pituitary body (Trendelenburg, 1926a). The distribution of the active principles between posterior, intermediate and anterior part was examined using histological techniques for the control of separation and bioassay for oxytocic, vasopressor, antidiuretic and melanophore-expanding activity (van Dyke, 1926). The first three were mainly found in the posterior lobe, while the melanophore-expanding activity was located chiefly in the intermediate lobe. The presence in the cerebro-spinal fluid of oxytocic, vasopressor and antidiuretic activity was established, and it was found that these activities remained after total removal of the pituitary body (Sato, 1928). This led to the quantitative determination of active principles in the tuber cinereum and the observation that its content was higher than in other parts of the brain. Trendelenburg was fully cognizant of the general importance of this work when he concluded that the tuber cinereum exhibited functions of internal secretion (Trendelenburg and Sato, 1928). This was the first recognition of active principles of the pituitary as constituents of parts of the central nervous system. Although these principles were presumed at the time to be peptides, their chemical nature remained to be clarified by the work of du Vigneaud et al. (1953).

By the end of 1927 the manuscript of the first volume of the hormone book had been completed. It dealt with: sex glands and placenta, pituitary body, suprarenals and other chromaffin tissues. It was published in 1929 (Trendelenburg, 1929a). In the meantime Trendelenburg had moved to Berlin in the summer of 1927 where literary work and experimental studies continued on the topics encompassed by the second volume, e.g., thyroid, parathyroid, islets of Langerhans and insulin, thymus, epiphysis. In 1930 an acute illness slowed down Trendelenburg's work but the problems occupied him until close to his death early in 1931. Volume 2 of the hormone book was posthumously completed [by Otto Krayer] and published in 1934 (Trendelenburg, 1934).

All through his active life as an investigator Trendelenburg never lost interest in problems of the physiology and pharmacology of the circulation. During the three Berlin years the circulatory system received major attention in the department. Failure of the circulation caused by incompetence of the heart was more sharply than before distinguished from vascular failure owing mainly to inadequate venous return as, for instance, in circulatory failure from histamine in carnivorous animals (Rühl, 1930). Analeptics, such as pentylenetetrazol [Cardiazol®], were shown to have no direct effect upon the heart (Bülbring, 1930). They acted upon the circulation in failure by their central nervous system action, e.g. when respiration was depressed by morphine (Gremels, 1931) or when central vasomotor influences were diminished as in poisoning with barbiturates. Attention was also given during this time to new members of the epinephrine series, i.e., synephrine and neosynephrine [phenylephrine]. They had been prepared in the department by H. Legerlotz and the first studies on their cardiac and general circulatory action were carried out (Kuschinsky, 1930; Kuschinsky and Oberdisse, 1931). Trendelenburg (1930a) was impressed by the possibility that substances of this type might have a more favorable ratio between cardiac and peripheral circulatory action than epinephrine which often puts under exceptional stress a heart impaired in its function.

As the son of a surgeon, as an auxiliary surgeon himself at the end of World War One, and as the subject of several major surgical interventions because of a recurrent intestinal illness, Trendelenburg was deeply interested in the development of general anesthesia. Theoretically and experimentally it was more the way of how to conduct general anesthesia safely than the theory of general anesthesia which attracted his attention. It was general anesthesia utilizing the inhalation of gases or vapor which for him held the greatest promise. In this he was stimulated by the investigation of Haggard (1924, I–V) on ether. Trendelenburg stressed the importance of the concept of the "safe anesthetic concentration" of the gases and vapors. The future of general anesthesia, he believed, belongs to gases with adequate potency and relatively low solubility in blood and tissues, so that the safe anesthetic concentration of the gases may be used (together with an adequate oxygen supply) from the beginning to the end of the anesthetic procedure and that induction as well as recovery upon cessation of anesthesia will he fast. In a lecture before the surgical section of the 'assembly of scientists and physicians' Trendelenburg (1929b) formulated his ideas on the theory of anesthesia with gases. His call remained largely unheeded in Germany. However, Trendelenburg's pupil O. Krayer carried his thoughts to the USA where at Harvard Medical School they inspired the young surgeon H. K. Beecher later to initiate anesthesia as a separate discipline of surgery and the young pharmacologists A. Goldstein and D. S. Riggs who carried the ideas further.

His paper on the "theory of inducing anesthesia with gases" (Trendelenburg, 1929b) was a step in the direction towards that scientific human pharmacology which he deemed desirable. Quite early in his life he had asked himself whether the separation of pharmacology from the clinic (as instigated by Schmiedeberg) did not, in the long run, constitute a danger for the discipline of pharmacology. In 1929, at a meeting of the German Medical Society on diseases of the metabolism, he voiced his concern about the separation of theoretical from practical pharmacology as follows: "So, in all earnestness, it may be asked whether the time has arrived for removing the separation of pharmacotherapeutists into theoreticians and practitioners by, on the one hand, giving the theoretical pharmacologist access to the patient and, on the other hand, providing the young clinicians with the opportunity of penetrating more deeply into the problems of theoretical pharmacology than has been done over recent decades. Thus, the pharmacologist will again become familiar with the problems of the clinician of which today he knows too little; and the clinician will be able to prepare himself for the task of filling a vast gap, namely to develop Human Pharmacology " (Trendelenburg, 1930b).

[Krayer's manuscript ends here with the note "Arzneimittel-verordnungslehre here", a reference to Trendelenburg's highly successful guide, for students and physicians, to rational pharmacotherapy. While deliberately disregarding all theoretical aspects, the author presented, according to indications, information on reliable drugs, including their doses, their fate in the human body, their side effects and the dangers they might present. The first edition was published in 1926 (Trendelenburg, 1926b), followed by a second in 1929; the third, posthume, was edited by Otto Krayer 1931, who also took care of the fourth edition in 1938 – then working at the American University in Beirut. Two more editions followed during the war by Ludwig Lendle in 1944 and 1945, and the seventh edition in 1952 by Otto Krayer and Manfred Kiese.]

# *References*

BÜLBRING, E. (1930). Die Wirkung einiger neuerer Herzmittel am durchströmten Froschherz. Arch. exp. Path. Pharmakol.,152, 257-272.

BÜLBRING, E. (1931). Über die Beziehungen zwischen Epithelkörperchen, Calciumstoffwechsel und Knochenwachstum. Arch. exp. Path. Pharmakol., 162, 209-248.

COLLIP, J. B. (1925). The extraction of a parathyroid hormone which will prevent or control parathyroid tetany and which regulates the level of blood calcium. J. Biol. Chem., 63, 395-438.

DYKE, H. B. van (1926). Die Verteilung der wirksamen Stoffe der Hypophyse auf verschiedene Teile derselben. Arch. exp. Path. Pharmakol., 114, 262-274.

FRASER, Th. R. (1892). Strophanthus hispidus: its natural history, chemistry and pharmacology. Pharmacology: Trans. Roy. Soc. Edinburgh, 36, II, 343-457.

GREMELS, H. (1931). Über die Einwirkung einiger zentralerregender Mittel auf Atmung und Kreislauf. Arch. exp. Path. Pharmakol., 162, 29-45.

HAGGARD, H. W. (1924, I-V). The absorption, distribution and elimination of ethyl ether.
I. The amount of ether absorbed in relation to the concentration inhaled and its fate in the body. J. Biol. Chem., 59, 737-751.
II. Analysis of the mechanism of absorption and elimination of such a gas or vapor as ethyl ether. J. Biol. Chem., 59, 753-770.

III. The relation of the concentration of ether, or any similar volatile substance, in the central nervous system to the concentration in the arterial blood, and the buffer action of the body. J. biol. Chem., 59, 771-781.

IV. The anesthetic concentration of ether and the physiological response to various concentrations. J. biol. Chem., 59, 783-793.

V. The importance of the volume of breathing during the induction and termination of ether anesthesia. J. biol. Chem., 59, 795-802.

HEUBNER, W. (1931). Paul Trendelenburg. Klin. Wschr., 10, 479.

JANSSEN, S. & PIETRKOWSKI, G. (1931). Paul Trendelenburg. Münch. med. Wschr., 1931, 452-453.

KRAYER, O. (1928). Über Verteilung und Ausscheidunng des Jodes nach Zufuhr von Schilddrüsenstoffen. Arch. exp. Path. Pharmakol., 128, 116-125.

KRAYER, O. (1931). Paul Trendelenburg 24.III.1884 – 4.II.1931. Arch. exp. Path. Pharmakol., 102, II-III.

KÜHL, G. (1927). Untersuchung zur Hormonwirkung der Nebennierenrinde. Pflügers Arch. ges. Physiol., 215, 277-290.

KUSCHINSKY, G. (1930). Untersuchungen über Sympatol, einen adrenalinähnlichen Körper. Arch. exp. Path. Pharmakol., 156, 290-308.

KUSCHINSKY, G. & OBERDISSE, K. (1931). Die Kreislaufwirkungen des Meta-Sympatols. Arch. exp. Path. Pharmakol., 162, 46-55.

LAEWEN, A. (1904). Quantitative Untersuchungen über die Gefäßwirkung von Suprarenin. Arch. exp. Path. Pharmakol., 51, 415-441.

LINDNER, J. (1957). Zeittafeln zur Geschichte der pharmakologischen Institute des deutschen Sprachgebietes. Aulendorf i. Württ.: Editio Cantor.

LOEWI, O. (1932). Eröffnungsansprache anläßlich der Tagung der Deutschen Pharmakologischen Gesellschaft 1932 in Wiesbaden. Arch. exp. Path. Pharmakol., 167, 17-18.

MAGNUS, R. (1904). Versuche am überlebenden Dünndarm von Säugetieren I. Mittheilung. Pflügers Arch. ges. Physiol., 102, 123-151.

RÜHL, A. (1930). Über Gefäßinsuffizienz. Arch. exp. Path. Pharmakol., 148, 24-55.

SATO, G. (1928). Über die Beziehungen des Diabetes insipidus zum Hypophysenhinterlappen und zum Tuber cinereum. Arch. exp. Path. Pharmakol., 131, 45-69.

SCHULTEN, H. (1925a). Zur Bestimmung der freien Ca-Ionen nach Brinkmann und van Dam. Biochem. Zeitschr., 164, 47-52.

SCHULTEN, H. (1925b). Das Hormon der Nebenschilddrüsen. Klin. Wschr., 4, 2487-2489.

SHIMIDZU, K. (1924). Versuche über die Steigerung der Adrenalinempfindlichkeit sympathisch innervierter Organe nach der Abtrennung von den zugehörigen Ganglien. Arch. exp. Path. Pharmakol., 104, 254-264.

STRAUB, W. (1931). Paul Trendelenburg †. Dtsch. med. Wschr., 57, 374-376.

STROOMANN, G. (1931). Paul Trendelenburg. Erg. Physiol., 32, 5-9.

TRENDELENBURG, P. (1909). Vergleichende Untersuchung über den Wirkungsmechanismus und die Wirkungsintensität glykositischer Herzgifte. Arch. exp. Path. Pharmakol., 61, 256-273.

TRENDELENBURG, P. (1910). Bestimmung des Adrenalingehaltes im normalen Blut sowie beim Abklingen der Wirkung einer einmaligen intravenösen Adrenalininjektion mittels physiologischer Meßmethode. Arch. exp. Path. Pharmakol., 63, 161-176.

TRENDELENBURG, P. (1912). Physiologische und pharmakologische Untersuchungen an der isolierten Bronchialmuskulatur. Arch. exp. Path. Pharmakol., 69, 79-107.

TRENDELENBURG, P. (1917). Physiologische und pharmakologische Versuche über die Dünndarmperistaltik. Arch. exp. Path. Pharmakol., 81, 57-129.

TRENDELENBURG, P. (1922). Über den Gehalt der Hypophysenhinterlappen-Extrakte an uteruserregenden Substanzen. Münch. med. Wschr., 4, 106-107.

TRENDELENBURG, P. (1923). Die Adrenalinsekretion unter normalen und gestörten Bedingungen. Erg. Physiol., 21, 500-557.

TRENDELENBURG, P. (1924). Adrenalin und adrenalinverwandte Substanzen. Heffters Handb. exp. Pharmakol., 2, 1130-1293, Berlin: Springer.

TRENDELENBURG, P. (1926a). Pharmakologie und Physiologie des Hypophysenhinterlappens. Erg. Physiol., 25, 364-438.

TRENDELENBURG, P. (1926b). Grundlagen der allgemeinen und speziellen Arzneiverordnung. Berlin: F.C.W. Vogel; 2 (Berlin); 3, 4 ed. O. Krayer (Berlin 1931, 1938); 5, 6 ed. L. Lendle (Berlin 1944, 1945); 7 ed. O. Krayer & M. Kiese (Berlin: Springer 1952).

TRENDELENBURG, P. (1929a). Die Hormone, ihre Physiologie und Pharmakologie, Vol. I. Berlin: Springer.

TRENDELENBURG, P. (1929b). Theorie des Narkotisierens mit Gasen. Narkose und Anaesthesie, 2, 1-12.

TRENDELENBURG, P. (1930a). Über die Kreislaufwirkung des Sympatols. Dtsch. med. Wschr., 56, 1987-1988.

TRENDELENBURG, P. (1930b). Kritik der Pharmakotherapie des Verdauungskanals. I. Pharmakologischer Teil. Verhandlg. Gesellsch. f. Verdauungs- und Stoffwechselkrankheiten, IX. Tagung in Berlin (16.-18. Okt. 1929), 37-45. Leipzig: Thieme.

TRENDELENBURG, P. (1934). Die Hormone, ihre Physiologie und Pharmakologie, Vol. II (ed.. Krayer, O.). Berlin: Springer.

TRENDELENBURG, P. & GOEBEL, W. (1921). Tetanie nach Entfernung der Epithelkörperchen und Calciummangel im Blute. Arch. exp. Path. Pharmakol., 89, 171-199.

TRENDELENBURG, P. & SATO, G. (1928). Über den Einfluß von Hypophyse und Tuber cinerium auf den Wasserhaushalt. Arch. exp. Path. Pharmakol., 128, 114.

VIGNEAUD, V. du, RESSLER, C., SWAN, J. M., ROBERTS, C. W., KATSOYANNIS, P. G. & GORDON, S. (1953) The synthesis of an octapeptide amide with the hormonal activity of oxytocin. J. Am. Chem. Soc., 75, 4879-4880.

August Wilhelm Forst

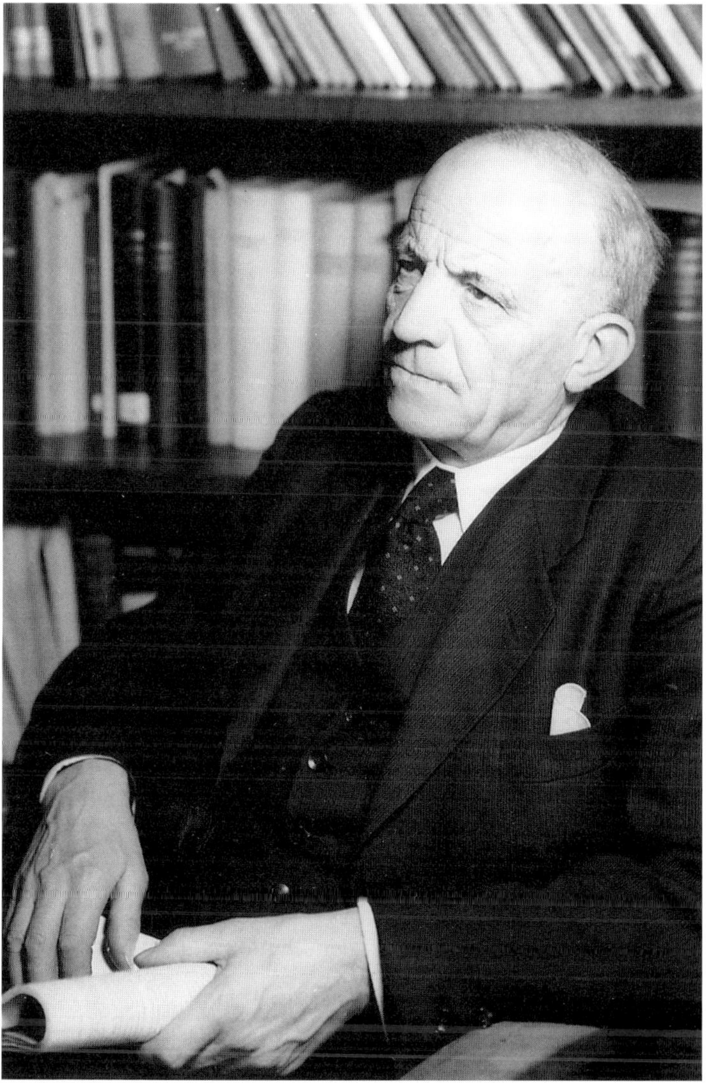

*August Wilhelm Forst*

# August Wilhelm Forst
# 1890 – 1981[*]

August Wilhelm Forst was born the son of the chemist Dr. phil. Karl Forst in Milano on June 10. 1890. His father was director of a local chemical factory. From 1894 the family lived in Frankfurt a. Main where Forst attended the Wöhler-Realgymnasium. After having finished school he read medicine, from 1909 to 1914, in Heidelberg, Freiburg and München. Under M. Borst in München he achieved the degree of Dr. med. in 1914; his thesis dealt with congenital varicose veins and originated from the Senckenbergian Institute of Pathological Anatomy in Frankfurt a. M. (Forst, 1915).

During the First World War Forst served as a medical officer of the mountain regiment. Thereafter he continued his studies in chemistry under Willstätter in München which he had already started before the war. He was promoted to Dr. phil. in March 1924 with a thesis on attempts to prepare beta-oxindole-propionic acid. From January 1924 he was an assistant of Walther Straub who, at the end of 1923, had become head of the Department of Pharmacology of the University of München. Under Straub he qualified as Lecturer in Pharmacology in 1928, with the thesis "On the detoxication of prussic acid" (Forst, 1928b). With the seizure of power by the National Socialists in 1933 Forst's academic career was interrupted. It was to Straub's credit that, notwithstanding the prevailing political climate, he offered Forst the opportunity in his department to develop into an independent scientist, although without any chance of a promotion. In this way, Forst was able to keep his family intact and to devote him-

---

[*] Biographical references: v. Werz, 1955; Lindner, 1957; Poggendorff, 1958; Halbach, 1960; Reiter, 1960; Braun, 1970; Forth, 1981; Dudel, 1982.

self to his work at the university. Shortly before the end of the Second World War and after the death of his mentor on October 22, 1944, the "Assistent" Forst was installed as the acting head of a department which had been largely destroyed in an air raid. In 1946 Forst was promoted to full professor in München and named director of the department, the reconstruction of which he skilfully carried through. Simultaneously he served as Dean of the Medical Faculty from 1946 to 1948. In 1951 he was elected a member of the Bavarian Academy of Sciences. Forst directed his department until 1961, and he died in München on August 4, 1981.

After having joined the Department of Pharmacology in München in 1924 Walther Straub suggested to him the development of a chemical method for the isolation of the uterine stimulant constituents of ergot. By the use of 50% acetone in water, it proved possible to extract quantitatively all water soluble and insoluble components from pulverized ergot, and then to separate the water insoluble alkaloids ergotamine and ergotoxin from the water soluble amines tyramine, histamine and acetylcholine (Forst, 1926a,b, 1936). In collaboration with H. Weese Forst determined by bioassay on the guinea-pig ileum the histamine content of various commercial preparations of ergot. They found large differences in the histamine content of different preparations, usually in inverse relation to their alkaloid content; hence, in some of these preparations an effect on the uterus could be expected to be in large part due to histamine (Forst and Weese, 1926).

In 1925, the health organisation section of the League of Nations organized in Geneva the second international conference on the biological standardization of certain drugs, under the chairmanship of H. H. Dale. On September 1, Straub as a member of this conference, reported Forst's method for the quantitative determination of the specific ergot alkaloids. Concerning the preparations of ergot, the original minutes of this meeting say: "The

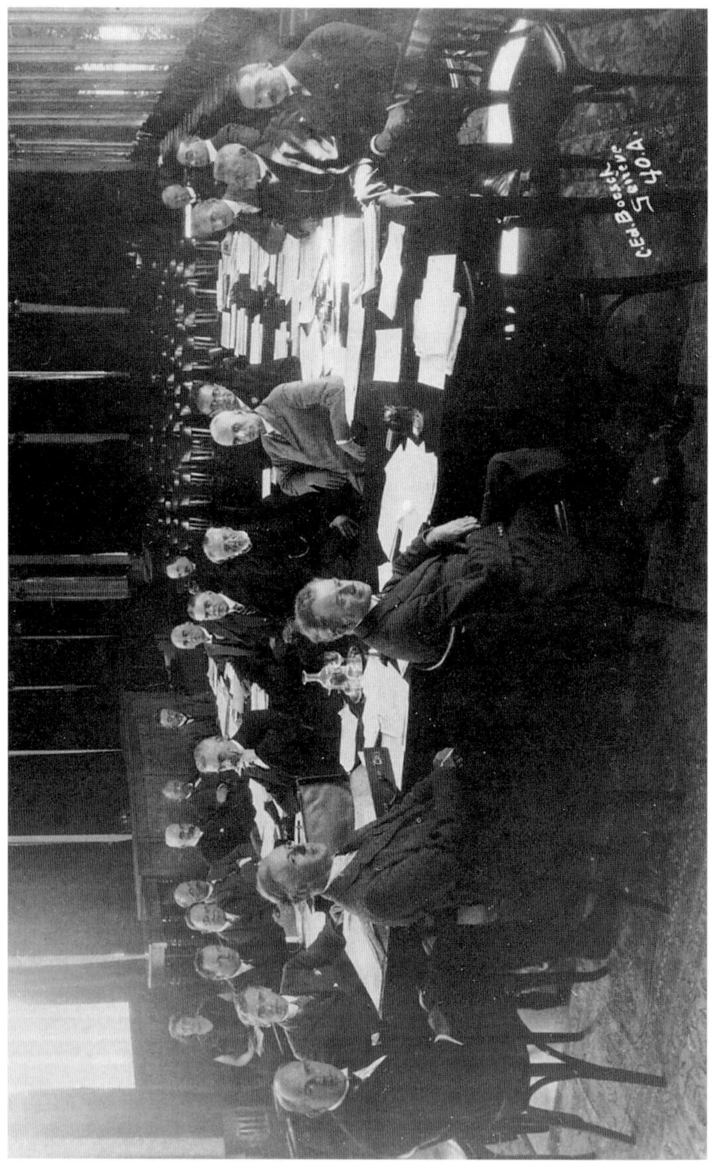

*La seconde Conférence internationale de la Société des Nations
pour la standardisation biologique de certains médicaments s'est réunie
à Genève, du 31 août au 3 septembre 1925.*

*Président: M. le docteur H.H. DALE.*

*MM. les professeurs:*

(1) *Dr. R. GAUTIER, Section d'hygiène de la Société des nations;*
(2) *Assistant de GAUTIER;*
(3) *C. VOEGTLIN, Washington;*
(4) *W. STRAUB, Munich;*
(5) *P. TRENDELENBURG, Fribourg en Br.;*
(6) *A. R. CUSHNY, Edimbourg;*
(7) *R. MAGNUS, Utrecht;*
(8) *A. KROGH, Copenhague;*
(9) *H. H. DALE (Londres);*
(10) *E. ROST, Berlin;*
(11) *E. POULSSON, Oslo;*
(12) *REID HUNT, Boston;*
(13) *J. J. R. MACLEOD, Toronto;*
(14) *H. H. MEYER, Vienne;*
(15) *E. v. KNAFFL-LENZ (Secrétaire), Vienne;*
(16) *C. W. EDMUNDS, Ann Arbor (Michigan);*
(17) *M. le professeur HEYMANS fils (Gand) assistait également aux séances;*
(18) *J. F. HEYMANS, Gand;*
(19) *W. KOLLE, Francfort s/M.;*
(20) *W. E. DIXON, Cambridge;*
(21) *M. TIFFENEAU, Paris;*
(a) *sténographe;*
(b) *traducteur.*

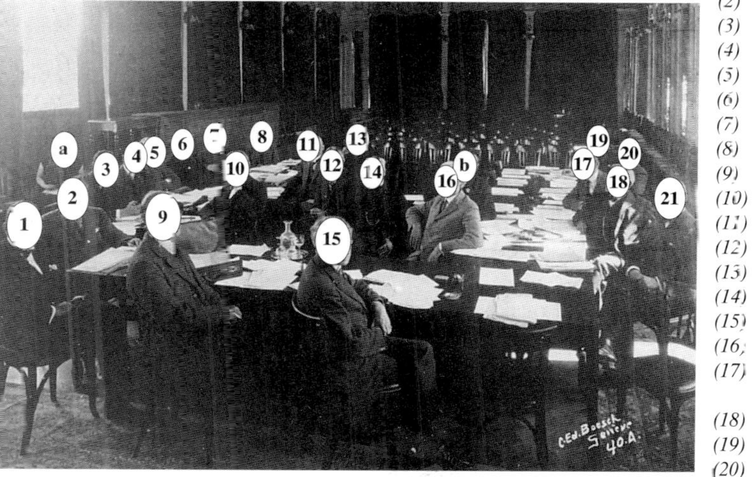

members of the Conference are of the opinion: That the question of the biological standardization of ergot is not yet ripe for final decision, and that it is desirable to give further study to the biological methods which have already been described, and to investigate those which may be discovered in the future, and especially to compare the results obtained by such methods with those obtained by the chemical method, presented to the Conference by Professor Straub" (Dale, 1925; Knaffl-Lenz, 1928; see picture of participants).

Forst conducted extensive studies on the detoxication of prussic acid (HCN) in mice, rats and rabbits. They revealed that – even after intoxication leading to loss of all reflexes – abolition of respiratory paralysis and reversal of all toxic symptoms could be rapidly achieved by the intravenous injection of dioxyacetone and colloidal sulphur. Complete recovery was obtained even after ten-fold the lethal dose of HCN was administered orally. Dioxyacetone was found to be beneficial with a rapid onset of effect on the medulla oblongata; it was also able to counteract the central respiratory paralysis induced by other agents. Colloidal sulphur, on the other hand, was responsible for the subsequent actual detoxication of HCN by the formation of rhodanid (Forst, 1928a,b; 1932). Later on Forst and Felix tested the view, occasionally expressed in the literature, that in the anacid stomach orally administered cyanides of alkali metals are less toxic (or are even devoid of toxicity) than solutions of HCN. However, when they used sodium bicarbonate to render the stomach contents of mice alkaline, the mean lethal dose of 9,9 µg/g KCN was the same as in controls without $NaHCO_3$ (Forst and Felix, 1953).

Forst was especially interested in checking experimentally old pharmacognosy reports on the effectiveness of various medicinal plants. Hence, he studied Lactuca virosa, the milk of which – when harvested during the blossoming period – is initially white but turns brown on drying and is then known as "lactucarium";

it then has the same colour as the milk of the poppy and shares with it a hypnotic effect. Forst isolated two active agents in crystalline form, the bitter and nitrogen-free substances lactucin and lactucopicrin. In order to demonstrate a sedative effect, he let mice move freely on a circular, smoked paper; in this way he was able to detect specific patterns of movement as well as the extent of their spontaneous mobility (Forst, 1937; 1938a,b). For quantitative measurements of spontaneous activity he used a suspended "running plate", the movements of which activated electrical contacts. He found that of the two bitter substances lactucin had the more potent sedative action (Forst, 1940). On behalf of the "Office International d'Hygiène Publique" in Paris, Forst compared with this method the central effect of dihydrodesoxymorphine sulphate with that of morphine; he found the former to be ten times more potent than morphine (Forst, 1939).

When Forst investigated the cardiovascular effects of extracts of the blossoms of Arnica montana in cats, he was the first to find evidence for relatively high concentrations of choline in the dried blossoms. On intravenous injection, the extracts – like choline – initially lowered the blood pressure, followed by a return to normal or even above the pre-injection level. The simple acetylation of the extracts by heating with acetic acid anhydride greatly increased their activity, indicating that choline rather than a labile choline ester was present. Simultaneously, H. Thies succeeded in demonstrating by chemical means the presence of choline in arnica extracts in the form of gold double salt (Forst, 1943a). When extracts were obtained with organic solvents in which choline is not soluble even as the free base, the results differed from those obtained with choline: after an initial fall in blood pressure a very pronounced pressor response and increase in heart rate was seen. This led to the supposition that the extracts of the blossoms of arnica montana contained not only choline but an additional substance with pronounced vasopressor and tachycardic effects. The ability of cocaine to increase its duration of action, and of ergotamine to abolish its pressor effect, are in favour of a vasopres-

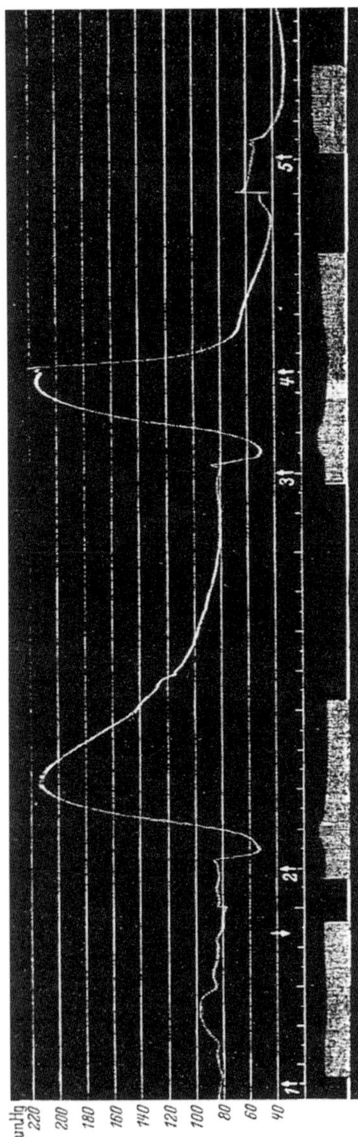



*Effect of choline and atropine on blood pressure and heart rate of a cat under chloralose. Recorded were (from top to bottom): blood pressure (with scale along ordinate), time (in min), heart rate (height of excursion of lever inversely proportional to frequency). Prior to onset of recording: 4 infusions of nicotine tartrate, 1%, 10 mg/kg, during 3 min 45 s each. At 1: the 5th infusion of nicotine. At 2, 3 and 5: 5mg/kg choline i.v. each. At 4: atropine, 2 mg/kg i.v. (Taken from Forst, 1943b, Fig.4).*

sor substance with sympathomimetic properties; however this substance was relatively unstable, and its structure remains to be elucidated (Forst, 1943a).

As Arnica montana contained choline, Forst became interested in investigating the ganglionic effects of this substance (1943b). Dale had attributed to choline two different types of action: a "muscarinic" depressor effect is antagonized by atropine, following which choline raises the blood pressure through a "nicotinic" effect; the latter is prevented by large doses of nicotine (Dale, 1914). Forst did not pretreat the animals with atropine and he studied the response to choline after ganglionic block by repeated injections of nicotine. He used purified nicotine so as to prevent the initial depressor effect of "aged" nicotine described in the literature. He recorded the blood pressure and the heart rate of cats and gave repeated injections of nicotine tartrate, until the pronounced initial pressor effect disappeared indicating ganglion blockade by nicotine. Thereafter choline caused a biphasic response: the initial depressor effect, accompanied by bradycardia, was followed by a rapid rise in blood pressure by 150 mm Hg together with an increase in heart rate. Identical responses to further injections of choline were obtained as soon as the blood pressure had returned to normal. However, an injection of atropine, given at the peak of the pressure response, immediately reduced the blood pressure to values below the pre-injection level; further injections of choline then exclusively lowered blood pressure and heart rate (see Figure). Prior removal of the adrenal glands failed to affect these responses. Thus, under these conditions the pressor response to choline revealed itself as a "muscarinic" rather than as a "nicotinic" effect. "Hence, the interpretation of the pressor response to choline as a nicotinic effect requires revision" (Forst, 1943b).

The finding that choline has a pressor effect even after blockade of the ganglionic nicotinic receptors and that this is abolished by atropine, was surprising in so far as it was irreconcilable with the then prevailing views concerning the receptors within autonomic ganglia. Dale's school tended to adhere to the assumption that the ganglia of the autonomic nervous system differed from e. g. smooth muscle cells in possessing exclusively nicotinic acetylcholine receptors. In view of today's knowledge, Forst's observations have to be interpreted as an early and clear pointer to the existence of muscarinic acetylcholine receptors on sympathetic ganglion cells. Why, then, did it take about 20 years until this concept was generally accepted? On the one hand, the timing of his publication just before the end of the Second World War was not conducive to a wide dissemination of these important findings. On the other hand, Forst shared the fate of his successors who found it very difficult to break out of the framework of the "doctrine" defined above. Thus, Forst (1943b), for instance, discussed an action of choline on peripheral sympathetic ganglion cells in the vessel wall, since – according to the "doctrine" – the pre- and paravertebral ganglia were blocked by nicotine. Even 13 years later U. Trendelenburg (1956) wrote in his summary: "It is suggested that the superior cervical ganglion of the cat possesses not only acetylcholine receptors but, in addition, separate receptors for histamine, for pilocarpine and for 5-HT"; the conclusion that there exist muscarinic ganglionic receptors was avoided by the postulate of "receptors for pilocarpine". It was only during the fifties and sixties that the "doctrine" was revised, by the cumulative weight of numerous reports demonstrating ganglion stimulating effects of pilocarpine and muscarine; hence, the existence of ganglionic muscarinic receptors was eventually accepted (see, for instance: Root, 1951; Trendelenburg, 1954; Ambache et al., 1956; Konzett and Waser, 1956; Jones, 1963). Electrophysiological (Eccles and Libet, 1961; Takeshige and Volle, 1962) and classical (Trendelenburg, 1966; Flacke and Gillis, 1968) methods finally showed that acetylcholine, released by preganglionic stimulation, could even result in muscarinic ganglionic transmission.

It was essential for Forst's observations that the administration of choline was preceded by repeated injections of nicotine. Without being aware of Forst's observations, Trendelenburg (1957) found that repeated injections of nicotine resulted not only in the well known ganglionic block, but additionally enhanced the sensitivity of the superior cervical ganglion to various "non-nicotinic" substances like pilocarpine, histamine and 5-hydroxy-tryptamine. Thus, in Forst's experiments this nicotine-induced enhancement of the ganglionic sensitivity is likely to have contributed to the appearance of muscarinic effects of choline on sympathetic ganglia.

A very different interaction of choline with the sympathetic innervation was observed in experiments with the pupil of the mouse after its sensitization by removal of the superior cervical ganglion (Forst and Deininger, 1952a). On intravenous administration the mydriatic effect of adrenaline was much stronger than that of noradrenaline. However, this quantitative difference largely disappeared when the effect of noradrenaline was enhanced by the simultaneous injection of choline or methionine. The authors concluded that injected noradrenaline was methylated by substances known to be methyl donors. Indeed, they demonstrated that the simultaneous administration of the non-selective methyl group acceptor tellurium (given as potassium tellurite) was able to prevent the choline- and methionine-induced potentiation of the effects of noradrenaline (Forst and Deininger, 1952b).

Forst was very conscientious in carrying out his teaching duties. In addition to lectures and demonstrations for medical students he insisted on giving the pharmacology lectures also for pharmacists and for students of the natural sciences. He also took the trouble to write a comprehensive review on bismuth for the Handbook of Experimental Pharmacology (Forst, 1935). The printing plates for his review on detoxication mechanisms (for a text- and handbook of physiological chemistry) fell victim to the destruction of Würzburg shortly before the end of the war. Instead of having his manuscript typeset again after the war, he decided on a completely new version to be written after his retirement. This resulted in a comprehensive review of 658 pages which begins with Baumann's discovery of the detoxication of phenol by sulphate 1876 in Strassburg and ends with the most recent reports then available to the author. It was published in 1966 and relates the turbulent development, during nearly a century, of our views on how the organism handles xenobiotics (Forst, 1966).

# *References*

AMBACHE, N., PERRY, W. L. M. & ROBERTSON, P. A. (1956). The effect of muscarine on perfused superior cervical ganglia of cats. Brit. J. Pharmacol., 11, 442-448.

BAUMANN, E. (1876). Über gepaarte Schwefelsäuren im Organismus. Plügers Arch., 13, 285-308.

BRAUN, H. (1970). Professor A. W. Forst zum 80. Geburtstag. Med. Mschr.,24, 282.

DALE, H. H. (1914). The action of certain esters and ethers of choline, and their relation to muscarine. J. Pharmacol. exp. Ther., 6, 147-190.

DALE, H. H. (1925). Deuxième Conférence Internationale pour la Standardisation Biologique de certain Médicaments: Rapport du Dr. H. H. Dale. Société des Nations. Genève: C. 532. M. 183. 1925. III., C.H. 350.

DUDEL, J. (1982). August Wilhelm Forst – 10.6.1890-4.8.1981. Jhrb. Bayer. Akademie d. Wissensch., München.

ECCLES, R. M. & LIBET, B. (1961). Origin and blockade of the synaptic responses of curarized sympathetic ganglia. J. Physiology, 157, 484-503.

FLACKE, W. & GILLIS, R. A. (1968). Impulse transmission via nicotinic and muscarinic pathways in the stellate ganglion of the dog. J. Pharmacol. exp. Ther., 163, 266-276.

FORST, A. W. (1915). Über kongenitale Varizen. Frankfurter Ztschr.f. Pathologie, 17, 137-157.

FORST, A. W. (1926a). Auswertung des Alkaloidanteils im Mutterkorn auf chemischem Wege. Verhdlg. Dt. Pharmakolog. Ges. 1925. Arch. exp. Path. Pharmakol., 111, 50.

FORST, A. W. (1926b). Über die uteruswirksamen Substanzen im Mutterkorn. Teil I. Arch. exp. Path. Pharmakol., 114, 125-136.

FORST, A. W. (1928a). Zur Entgiftung der Blausäure. Verhdlg. Dt. Pharmakol. Ges. 1927. Arch. exp. Path. Pharmakol., 128, 150-152.

FORST, A. W. (1928b). Zur Entgiftung der Blausäure. Arch. exp. Path. Pharmakol., 128, 1-66.

FORST, A. W. (1932). Zum Antagonismus Kohlehydrate – Blausäure. Arch. exp. Path. Pharmakol., 167, 108-111.

FORST, A. W. (1935). Wismut. in: Hdb. d. exp. Pharmakologie (Heffter, Heubner), 3, Teil 4, pp. 2249-2739. Berlin: Springer.

FORST, A. W. (1936). Eine einfache, schonende Methode zur Isolierung des Alkaloidkomplexes aus dem Mutterkorn. Arch. exp. Path. Pharmakol., 181, 180.

FORST, A. W. (1937). Der Giftlattich, eine vergessene Heilpflanze. München. med. Wschr., 84, 1251-1254.

FORST, A. W. (1938a). Neue Wege zur Erkennung sedativer Wirkung. Arch. exp. Path. Pharmakol., 189, 288-297.

FORST, A. W. (1938b). Demonstration einer Apparatur zur Messung sedativer Wirkung. Verhdlg. Dt. Pharmakolog. Ges. 1938. Arch. exp. Path. Pharmakol., 190, 231.

FORST, A. W. (1939). Morphin und Dihydrodesoxymorphin, verglichen mittels einer neuen Methode der Motilitätsmessung. Arch. exp. Path. Pharmakol., 192, 257-270.

FORST, A. W. (1940). Pharmakologische Untersuchungen über die Lactuca virosa. Arch. exp. Path. Pharmakol., 195, 1-25.

FORST, A. W. (1943a). Zur Wirkung der Arnica montana auf den Kreislauf. Arch. exp. Path. Pharmakol., 201, 242-260.

FORST, A. W. (1943b). Zur Wirkung von gereinigtem Nicotin und von Cholin auf den Kreislauf. Arch. exp. Path. Pharmakol., 201, 261-277.

FORST, A. W. (1966). Entgiftung. In: Physiologische Chemie (Hrsg. B. Flaschenträger & E. Lehnartz), 2, 2. Teil – Bandteil d/alpha, pp. 1-658 and VIII – XXX. Berlin-Heidelberg-New York: Springer.

FORST, A. W. & DEININGER, R. (1952a). Die denervierte Mäusepupille als Testobjekt für Adrenalin. Arch. exp. Path. Pharmakol., 215, 354-362.

FORST, A. W. & DEININGER, R. (1952b). Die Methylierung des Noradrenalins durch Acetylcholin. Arch. exp. Path. Pharmakol., 215, 378-388.

FORST, A. W. & FELIX, W. (1953). Vergiftung mit Alkalizyanid bei anacidem Magen. Z. Biol., 106, 77-80.

FORST, A. W. & WEESE, H. (1926). Über die uteruswirksamen Substanzen im Mutterkorn – II. Teil: Histamin. Arch. exp. Path. Pharmakol., 117, 232-239.

FORTH, W. (1981). August Wilhelm Forst, 1890-1981. München. med. Wschr., 123, 56.

HALBACH, H. (1960). Zum 70. Geburtstag von Prof. Dr. med. et phil. A. W. Forst. München. med. Wschr., 102, 1363-64.

JONES, A. (1963). Ganglionic actions of muscarinic substances. J. Pharmacol. exp. Ther., 141, 195-205.

KNAFFL-LENZ, E. (1928). Bericht über die Arbeiten und Vorschläge der internationalen Konferenzen, welche von der Hygieneorganisation des Völkerbundes behufs Vereinheitlichung der biologischen Wertbestimmung von Heilmitteln veranstaltet wurden. Arch. exp. Path. Pharmakol., 135, 259-332.

KONZETT, H. & WASER, P. G. (1956). Zur ganglionären Wirkung von Muscarin. Helv. Physiol. Acta, 14, 202-206.

LINDNER, J. (1957). Zeittafeln zur Geschichte der pharmakologischen Institute des deutschen Sprachgebietes. Aulendorf i. Württ.: Editio Cantor.

POGGENDORFF, J. C. (1958). Forst, August Wilhelm. Biogr.-Liter. Hdwrtb., VIIa, Teil 2.

REITER, M. (1960). Zum 70. Geburtstag von Professor Dr. Dr. A. W. Forst. Arzneim.-Forsch. (Drug Res.), 10, 489-490.

ROOT, M. A. (1951). Certain aspects of the vasopressor action of pilocarpine. J. Pharmacol. exp. Ther., 101, 125-131.

TAKESHIGE, C. & VOLLE, R. L. (1962). Bimodel response of sympathetic ganglia to acetylcholine following eserine or repetitive preganglionic stimulation. J. Pharmacol. exp. Ther., 138, 66-73.

TRENDELENBURG, U. (1954). The action of histamine and pilocarpine on the superior cervical ganglion and the adrenal glands of the cat. Brit. J. Pharmacol., 9, 481-487.

TRENDELENBURG, U. (1956). Modification of transmission through the superior cervical ganglion of the cat. J. Physiology, 132, 529-541.

TRENDELENBURG, U. (1957). Reaktion sympathischer Ganglien während der Ganglienblockade durch Nicotin. Arch. exp. Path. Pharmakol., 230, 448-456.

TRENDELENBURG, U. (1966). Transmission of preganglionic impulses through the muscarinic receptors of the superior cervical ganglion of the cat. J. Pharmacol. exp. Ther., 154, 426-440.

WERZ, R. v. (1955). Zum 65. Geburtstag von Professor Dr. A. W. Forst. Arzneim.-Forsch.(Drug Res.), 5, 353-354.

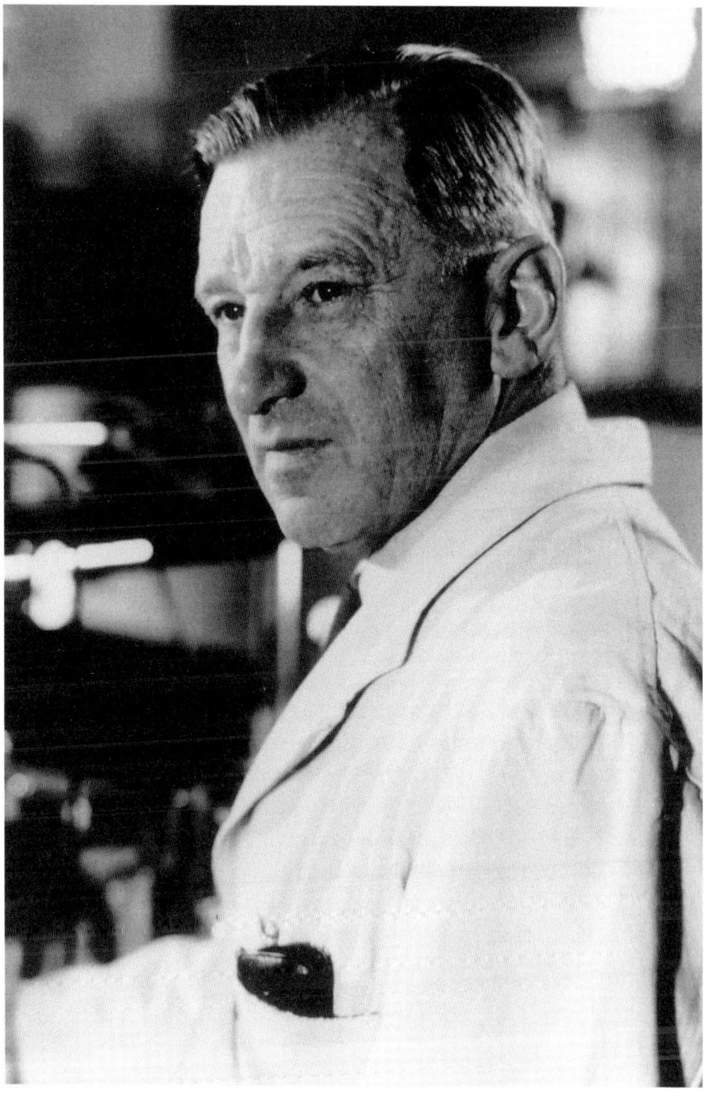

*Hellmut Weese*

# Hellmut Weese
# 1897 – 1954 *

Hellmut Weese was born in München on March 18, 1897. He was the son of the Lecturer in the History of Art Dr. Arthur Weese who, in 1906, moved to Switzerland, having been offered a position at the University of Bern. After completing his schooling in Bern Weese was inducted into the German Army in 1916 and took part in the First World War until 1918. From 1919 onwards he studied medicine at the Universities of Bern, Zürich and finally München, where he was licenced as a physician in 1924 and where he was awarded the degree of Dr. med. in 1925, with a thesis on the genesis of carcino-sarcomas. After a short period of clinical work in the Surgical Policlinic (under v. Redwitz) and in the Medical Hospital (under v. Romberg), in October 1925, Weese became an assistant of Walther Straub who, in 1923, had assumed the Directorship of the Department of Pharmacology of the University of München.

Already in 1928 Weese was promoted to Lecturer in Pharmacology, following studies on a novel analysis of the binding of digitalis glycosides by means of the heart-lung preparation of the cat. In 1929 Weese accepted an offer from the Farbenfabriken Bayer AG and assumed the direction of the Pharmacological Laboratories in Wuppertal-Elberfeld, as the successor to Fritz Eichholtz. In 1930 he became Lecturer in Pharmacology at the University of Köln and became professor there in 1936.

In 1939, at the beginning of the Second World War, Weese was inducted into the army as an advisory pharmacologist but

---

* Biographical sources: Corsten, 1938; Brücke, 1954; Hahn, 1954; Hecht and Schulemann, 1954; Killian, 1954, 1966; Lendle, 1954; Lindner, 1957; Poggendorff, 1960; Schadewaldt and Morich, 1990.

returned to Elberfeld in 1941. At the end of the war in 1945 and in addition to his scientific acitivities he assumed the position of a town councillor of the city of Elberfeld. In the spring of 1946 he was offered the chair of pharmacology at the Medical Academy of Düsseldorf. He accepted the position in addition to the directorship of the laboratories in Elberfeld so as to further the rebuilding of the university department. In 1948 and 1949 Weese also served as 'Prorektor' of the Düsseldorf Academy which was then in a deplorable condition. Afterwards he resigned as head of the university department to concentrate on his activities in Elberfeld. In January 1954, while removing a piece of apparatus from a cupboard of his laboratories in Elberfeld, Weese fell from a ladder and suffered a basal skull fracture; he died five days later, without regaining consciousness, on January 24, 1954.

As Straub's assistant, Weese began to extend Straub's studies of the action of digitalis glycosides on the frog isolated heart to the mammalian heart. For this purpose he used Starling's heart-lung preparation (HLP), adapted to the cat heart. He found that the doses of digitoxin and ouabain, which caused systolic arrest of the heart, amounted to only a fraction (6% and 9%, respectively) of the minimal lethal doses determined by Hatcher and Brody (1910) after intravenous infusions into cats. This indicated that, in the intact organism, organs other than the heart were also able to store digitalis glycosides (Weese, 1928). He studied the binding by various organs (kidney, liver, skeletal muscle) by including these organs into the HLP and by determining the cardiac toxicity after the glycoside had first passed the organ. Binding by the kidneys was equivalent to that of the heart, while much less binding was observed in liver and skeletal muscle, and lungs and blood bound no glycoside. Hence, despite the lower binding capacity, due to their abundant mass the other organs caused much more pronounced binding of the glycoside than the heart itself (Weese, 1929).

Although new duties awaited him in the Elberfeld laboratories, Weese was able to continue his experiments on the action of digi-

talis. In studies on the mechanism of the cumulative effect of digitoxin on the heart he re-examined the role of the aglycone digitoxigenin released (according to reports in the literature) from
digitoxin bound to non-cardiac tissue. However, his experiments
with the HLP revealed that the blood of digitalized cats contained no functionally demonstrable digitoxigenin and he concluded that the cumulative effect on the heart was due solely to
glycoside bound in the heart. This conclusion was supported by
further experiments in which cats received 50% of the minimal
lethal dose. Two to twelve days later the HLP was set up from
these animals and the isolated hearts received successive injections of digitoxin until cardiac arrest ensued. As the lowest dose
of digitoxin resulting in cardiac arrest was known (Weese, 1928),
the acutely administered amount of the glycoside represented
the complementary dose, in addition to the amount of digitoxin
left in the heart from the initial administration. The rate of the
decline of the glycoside left in heart proved to be constant with
time. The daily loss of the minimal lethal dose amounted to 3–4%;
hence, it took this dose of digitoxin about four weeks to disap-
pear from the heart (Weese, 1930).

Quasi-therapeutic effects of non-toxic doses of digitoxin were
demonstrable in the HLP when the arterial resistance was
increased stepwise until insufficiency resulted: up to the third day
after the administration of digitoxin, the hearts from treated cats
were less easily fatigued and remained functionally intact for
longer than those from animals not injected with the glycoside
(Weese and Dieckhoff, 1934).

A prerequisite for the exact measurement of cardiac performance in the HLP was the accurate recording of the rate of flow
on the arterial side of the artificial circulation. In the absence of
any adequate device Weese developed in the pharmacological
laboratories at Bayer "a mechanical, automatic flowmeter for a
closed circuit"; this was built by Karl Heuwing, in the workshop
of Straub's department in München (Weese, 1932a). The 'Weese

Stromuhr' was successful not only in his own hands but also in those of other experts of the HLP (for instance: Krayer and Mendez, 1942; Farah and Maresh, 1948; Brücke, 1954; Hawkins, Uhle and Krayer, 1964).

When discussing therapeutic problems with clinicians, Weese noticed "how little even scientifically oriented clinicians know of the new experimental results concerning the problems of digitalis glycosides". He saw a "deplorable gulf between the experimentalist and the clinician" which induced him to write the monograph "Digitalis", completed in October 1935 (Weese, 1936). Weese aimed at a consistent representation of the results of contemporary research "as a basis for future studies and clinical decisions in all questions pertaining to digitalis". For the required breadth of the treatment of this topic, especially of related areas, he was advised and helped by specialists, partly from the company in Elberfeld. In his final chapter on the treatment of patients with digitalis he was advised by the then most knowledgeable experts on cardiac insufficiency, Albert Fraenkel and Ernst Edens. Weese dedicated his monograph to Walther Straub; the book was widely acclaimed and became a standard text of lasting value.

Subsequently, Weese, together with Ernst Edens, wrote a monograph on the "Drug Treatment of Irregular Cardiac Activity", to which he contributed introductory chapters on the pathophysiology and pharmacology of cardiac arrhythmias as well as a chapter on their pharmacotherapy (Edens and Weese, 1944).

Weese's new field of activity, namely as a pharmacologist in the pharmaceutical industry who takes an integral role in the search for new drugs appeared to agree fully with his nature and his inclinations. His initiative and methodological independence and his devotion to careful experimentation and analysis, combined with a selfcritical and creative imagination, represented ideal prerequisites for his success.

Weese carried out a pharmacological analysis of barbituric acids alkylated on the nitrogen and found that the N-methylated homologue of phenobarbitone [Luminal®], methylphenobarbitone, retained full antiepileptic activity yet clearly had less hypnotic activity than phenobarbitone; hence, it had advantages when used clinically as an antiepileptic drug (Weese, 1932b). For several decades it has been in therapeutic use under the trade name Prominal®.

Even more significant were Weese's studies with the N-methylated barbiturate hexobarbitone, a homologue of cyclobarbitone [Phanodorm®], which made history under the name of Evipan®. In contrast to the then available hypnotics, i.e., the long acting diethylbarbituric acid, barbitone [Veronal®] and the hypnotics cyclobarbitone and phenobarbitone, hexobarbitone turned out to have a rapid onset and short duration of action; it could be considered to be "a true hypnotic for the rapid induction of sleep, relatively non-toxic and with a high therapeutic index" (Weese and Scharpff, 1932).

When mice or cats were injected intravenously with hypnotic doses of the readily soluble sodium salt of hexobarbitone, the animals became fully anaesthetized during the injection and recovered within about 30 min. Such observations induced Weese to propose that "Evipan® sodium could be useful as an injectable drug leading to shortlasting anaesthesia". The analysis of detailed animal experiments carried out to profile the sodium salt of Evipan® as an injectable short acting anaesthetic revealed that it could replace the then conventional very brief administration of ether, by providing anaesthesia of 5–15 min duration with minimal mental trauma to the patient (Weese, 1933a,b).

While clinical experience quickly confirmed that orally administered Evipan® was a reliable hypnotic, there were serious reservations to Weese's suggestion that injections of Evipan® sodium should be used to induce anaesthesia. We owe it to Weese's persistence and persuasiveness that he, together with his coworkers in Elberfeld and supportive clinicians, eventually overcame these difficulties. Hence, Hellmut Weese became the undeniable instigator of modern intravenous anaesthesia. He found international recognition when the committee of the International Anaesthesia Congress in New York in 1938 awarded him honorary membership.

The rapid onset and the short duration of action of hexobarbitone are due to its high lipid solubility; this ensures rapid passage through the blood-brain barrier as well as rapid redistribution within the organism. Other researchers soon found other barbiturates with similar pharmacological and physicochemical properties. Some had even higher lipid solubility, such as thiopentone [Pentothal®], and proved to have certain advantages over hexobarbitone. Weese also tried to improve his Evipan® and developed another thiobarbiturate with the provisional name 'Narkogen'. In animal experiments and in a large number of clinical administrations, 'Narkogen' was proven to be equal to thiopenthone (Weese and Koss, 1954); however, the compound was never marketed because of patent problems (Killian, 1966).

Whilst collaborating with surgeons to define appropriate modalities for the use of Evipan® sodium for the induction of anaesthesia, Weese took part in developing the new technique of 'combination anaesthesia'. He was particularly concerned about the training of 'anaesthetists', the specialists so badly needed by the clinics. In his lecture "Fundamental and Pharmacological Aspects of Modern Techniques of Anaesthesia" at the session 'Modern techniques of Anaesthesia' of a Congress of the German Surgical Society he stated: "Anglo Saxon countries are more progressive and more experienced than we are with respect to all techniques of anaesthesia, except peridural anaesthesia". He pointed out that from 1947 to 1949 the use of intravenous anaesthesia at the Mayo Clinic increased from 33% to 60%. He concluded his talk with the appeal: "Such statistics demonstrate unequivocally the progress made possible by the specialization of anaesthetists. The urgent need to also train here specialized anaesthetists with thorough theoretical knowledge and broad practical experience has long been common knowledge. May today's session bring to life the specialized anaesthetist and enable us to provide anaesthesia to patients as safely and with the variety of techniques available in other countries" (Weese, 1951a).

His persistent endeavours to improve anaesthesiology in Germany eventually led to the foundation of the German Society for Anaesthesia in München in 1953. Weese was awarded honorary membership of this society, "since he, like no other, had fought for the recognition of anaesthesiology as a speciality, against major resistance" (Killian, 1954).

Weese's appointment as an advisory pharmacologist to the army at the beginning of the Second World War represented a special challenge. He soon realized that the treatment of injured soldiers in field hospitals was deficient, especially with respect to the therapy of blood loss and shock. In 1939, in addition to fresh whole blood for transfusions, only stored citrated blood and crystalloid solutions were available for the treatment of blood loss and shock. However, transfusion of human blood turned out to be impractical, especially when many injured people had to be dealt with.

For Weese the treatment of blood loss and shock was primarily a haemodynamic problem; after an acute loss of blood, 50 to 70% of the physiological number of erythrocytes suffices to satisfy normal oxygen consumption, provided the lost plasma volume is quickly and permanently replaced. Hence, consideration of the blood volume is of paramount importance in the treatment of blood loss, shock and collapse. Intravenous infusions of physiological salt solutions leave the blood vessels within, at most, two hours, since, as Starling's studies showed, the fluid exchange between the circulation and the organs depends on the ratio between blood pressure and osmotic pressure of the plama (Starling, 1896).

"What we obviously lacked at the beginning of the war was an adequate colloidal solution for the treatment of blood loss of medium severity, of shock and of protoplasmatic collapse. The situation was similar to that in the First World War. It was Bayliss (1916) who then discovered a suitable colloid, gum arabic" (Weese, 1944). After considerations by the British 'shock commission' Bayliss was the first to reach the right conclusion from Starling's observations and to replace crystalloid solutions by a colloidal solution of gum arabic in the treatment of blood loss and shock. In the First World War "gum saline" was highly successful in spite of certain side effects.

The German side, on the other hand, failed to reach the same conclusion. Hence, it faced the same situation in 1939 as the British 'shock commission' did in 1916. Weese regarded it as his task to develop as quickly as possible a colloidal solution which was as useful a fluid replacement as was the 6% gum solution used by all armies of the Allies in the Second World War. Since gum powder was not available in Germany, a new colloid had to be found. Weese and his coworkers began their search in January 1940. Failures with biological colloids, which turned out to be chemically labile or easily degradable by enzymes or by oxidation, resulted in a search for the simplest possible, chemically neutral colloids. Before the end of 1940 they selected polyvinylpyrrolidone, 'Kollidon', which was a product of 'Reppe-Chemie' of BASF Ludwigshafen. In acute and chronic animal experiments this colloid proved the least toxic and fulfilled all expectations. Structurally 'Kollidon' resembles proteins but without the chemical reactivity of a protein. For fluid replacement they selected a polymer of an average molecular weight of 50,000. The 3.5% solution developed an osmotic pressure of about 400 mm water. 'Kollidon' is effective for 1–2 days, i.e., a concentration in the circulation is maintained which increases plasma volume. After three weeks it is no longer demonstrable in the organism. Blood clotting is unaffected. 'Kollidon' was then the first substance of non-animal origin which, like the serum proteins, served as a vehicle, i.e., it bound vitamins, hormones and drugs to release them where needed (Hecht and Weese, 1943).

Mass production of 'Kollidon', now introduced under the name of Periston® in ampoules of 500 ml, began in 1942. "Up to May 1944 more than 100,000 litres of Periston had been used to treat blood loss, shock and collapse, and hardly any shivering fit or other side effect has been observed. Thus, as far as compatibility is concerned, it is far superior to protein solutions or gum saline. In its clinical effectiveness (as in animal experiments), it is equivalent to solutions prepared from blood" (Weese, 1944). By 1950 infusions of Periston had been administered about one million times (Weese, 1951b). "There can be no doubt that thousands of injured soldiers of the Second World War owe their life to Weese's development of Periston (polyvinylpyrrolidone)" (Brücke, 1954). In recognition of his successful work on plasma expanders, Weese was made a member of the German Academy of Natural Scientists (Leopoldina) in Halle in 1943.

After the war, others developed a further plasma expander, dextran, which was produced by partial hydrolysis of bacterially synthesized glucopolysaccharide. Weese found that the haemodynamic effects of dextran were basically similar to those of 'Kollidon' (Weese, 1951b, 1953). However, 'Kollidon' differed from dextran in possessing the ability, if low molecular polyvinylpyrrolidone is used, to absorb reversibly certain substances which were then eliminated by the kidneys. For this purpose, 'Kollidon' of an average molecular weight of 20,000, named Periston N®, was produced of which between 75% and 100% is eliminated in the urine in 24 hours (Weese and Scholtan, 1951; Weese, 1953).

Weese was invited by Hans Killian, the former director of the Surgical University Hospital in Breslau, to co-edit a handbook "Die Narkose", which represented a total revision of Killian's monograph "Anaesthesia During Surgery", first published in 1934. Weese contributed the chapters on gas exchange, theory of

intravenously induced anaesthesia, the pharmacology of pheno-
thiazines, ganglionic blockade and barbiturates. After Weese's
death the publication of this book of more than 1,000 pages was
made possible in 1954 thanks to the help of his co-worker and
successor in Elberfeld, Wolfgang Wirth (Killian and Weese, 1954).

# *References*

BAYLISS, W. M. (1916). Methods of raising a low arterial pressure. Proc. Roy.
Soc. B., 89, 380-393.

BRÜCKE, F. (1954). Prof. Dr. H. Weese †. Österr. Chemiker-Ztg., 55, 88-89.

CORSTEN, II. (1938). Das Schrifttum der zur Zeit an der Universität Köln
wirkenden Dozenten. 137-138, Köln.

EDENS, E. & WEESE, H. (1944). Die medikamentöse Behandlung der unre-
gelmäßigen Herztätigkeit. Leipzig: S. Hirzel.

FARAH, A. & MARESH, G. (1948). Determination of the therapeutic, irre-
gularity, and lethal doses of cardiac glycosides in the heart-lung preparation
of the dog. J. Pharmacol. exp. Ther., 92, 32-42.

HAHN, F. (1954). Professor Dr. Hellmut Weese. Die Medizinische Nr. 12: 402.

HATCHER, R. A. & BRODY, J. G. (1910). The biological standardization of
drugs. Amer. J. Pharmacy, 82, 360-372.

HAWKINS, D. F., UHLE, F. C. & KRAYER, O. (1964). Studies on Veratrum
Alkaloids XXXVII. Chronotropic cardiac action and toxicity of N-alkyl
derivatives of veratramine. J. Pharmacol. exp. Ther., 145, 275-285.

HECHT, G. & SCHULEMANN, W. (1954). In memoriam Hellmut Weese. Arzneim.-Forsch. (Drug Res.),4, 218-220.

HECHT, G. & WEESE, H. (1943). Periston, ein neuer Blutflüssigkeitsersatz.
München. med. Wschr., 90, 11-15.

KILLIAN, H. (1954). Hellmut Weese †. Der Anästhesist, 3, 97-98.

KILLIAN, H. (1966). Das Abenteuer der Narkose. Erfahrungen und Erlebnisse
aus 40 Jahren Narkoseforschung. Tübingen: Grabert.

KILLIAN, H & WEESE, H. (1954). Die Narkose. Ein Lehr- und Handbuch.
XXVIII u. 1,003 pp., Stuttgart: Thieme.

KRAYER, O. & MENDEZ, R. (1942). Studies on Veratrum Alkaloids I. The
action of veratrine upon the isolated mammalian heart. J. Pharmacol. exp.
Ther., 74, 350-364.

LENDLE, L. (1954). Zum Gedächtnis von Hellmut Weese. Dtsch. med. Wschr.,
79, 447-448.

LINDNER, J. (1957). Zeittafeln zur Geschichte der pharmakologischen Institute des deutschen Sprachgebietes. Aulendorf i Württ.: Editio Cantor.

POGGENDORFF, J. C. (1960). Weese, Hellmut Ernst Richard Karl. Biogr.-Liter. Hdwrtb., VIIa Teil 4.

SCHADEWALDT, H. & MORICH, F.-J. (1990). 100 Jahre Pharmakologie bei Bayer 1890 – 1990. Leverkusen: Bayer AG.

STARLING, E. H. (1896). On the absorption of fluids from the connective tissue spaces. J. Physiology, 19, 312-326.

WEESE, H. (1928). Digitalisverbrauch und Digitaliswirkung im Warmblüter. I: Die Effektivdosen verschiedener Digitalisglykoside für das Herz. Arch. exp. Path. Pharmakol., 135, 228-244.

WEESE, H. (1929). Digitalisverbrauch und Digitaliswirkung im Warmblüter. II: Der extrakardiale Digitalisverbrauch und die Bedingungen der Glykosidbindung am Herzen. Arch. exp. Path. Pharmakol., 141, 329-350.

WEESE, H. (1930). Digitalisverbrauch und Digitaliswirkung im Warmblüter. III: Zur Entstehung der Kumulation. Arch. exp. Path. Pharmakol., 150, 14-20.

WEESE, H. (1932a). Eine mechanische, automatisch registrierende Stromuhr für den geschlossenen Kreislauf. Arch. exp. Path. Pharmakol., 166, 392-394.

WEESE, H. (1932b). Zur Pharmakologie des Prominal. Dtsch. med. Wschr., 58, 696.

WEESE, H. (1933a). Pharmakologie des intravenösen Kurznarkotikums Evipan-Natrium. Dtsch. med. Wschr., 59, 47-48.

WEESE, H. (1933b). Aus der Entwicklung der Schlafmittelsynthese. Medizin und Chemie, 1, 190-197.

WEESE, H. (1936). Digitalis. 296 pp., Leipzig: Thieme.

WEESE, H. (1944). Blutersatzprobleme. Med. Ztschr., 1, 19-23.

WEESE, H. (1951a). Moderne Betäubungsverfahren. Grundsätzliches und Pharmakologisches zu den modernen Anästhesieverfahren. Langenbecks Arch. u. Dtsch. Z. Chir., 267 (Kongreßbericht), 215-230.

WEESE, H. (1951b). Indifferente Kolloide in Chirurgie und innerer Medizin. Dtsch. med. Wschr., 76, 757-761.

WEESE, H. (1953). Therapeutische Möglichkeiten mit Blutersatzstoffen. München. med. Wschr., 95, 456-459.

WEESE, H. & DIECKHOFF, J. (1934). Zur Kumulation der Digitalisglykoside. Arch. exp. Path. Pharmakol., 176, 274-282.

WEESE, H. & KOSS, F. H. (1954). Über ein neues Ultrakurznarkotikum. Dtsch. med. Wschr., 79, 601-604.

WEESE, H. & SCHARPFF, W. (1932). Evipan, ein neuartiges Einschlafmittel. Dtsch. med. Wschr., 58, 1205-1207.

WEESE, H. & SCHOLTAN, W. (1951). Pharmakologie des Periston N. Dtsch. med. Wschr., 76, 1492-1493.

# Main Research Work of Otto Krayer
# 1899 – 1982

## *Thyroid hormones*

The earliest experimental work dealt with the function of the thyroid gland. The claims for an increase in the responsiveness of autonomic effector organs to physiological or pharmacological stimuli, based on the acute administration of thyroglobulin or thyroxin, were critically examined and could not be supported. The responses to epinephrine of blood pressure, of isolated segments of the amphibian and mammalian circulatory system, and of isolated segments of mammalian small intestine were investigated, as was the secretion of the cat submaxillary gland in vivo caused by nerve stimulation (Krayer and Sato, 1928). A study of the distribution and fate of iodine, in mammals, after administration of thyroglobulin or thyroxin revealed passage of a large proportion of their iodine into the bile. Biological experiments (metamorphosis of axolotl) established that some of the iodine-containing substances in bile retained characteristic thyroid activity (Krayer, 1928).

## *Pharmacology of the circulatory system.*
## *Studies on the failing heart*

Interest in cardiovascular physiology and pharmacology led to the acquisition of the techniques for the physiological analysis of site and mechanism of drug action. The technique of the heart-lung preparation of the dog, as developed by E. H. Starling, became of special importance. The methods were used, e.g., for the analysis of the circulatory effects of oxidized neoarsphen-aminc, which leads to a failure of the circulation by actions upon the vessels of the heart and lungs (Krayer, 1929, 1930); and for the elucidation of the actions of Kallikrein which are essentially due to vasodilatation (Krayer and Rühl, 1931). The versatility of the heart-lung preparation made possible the investigation, in the normal and failing heart, of the influence upon cardiac output of alterations of blood supply, arterial resistance, and heart rate and the study of the action of drugs under controlled conditions of heart failure (Krayer, 1931).

## *Neuro-humoral transmission in the mammalian heart*

A decade after the discovery of neuro-humoral vagal transmission in the frog heart by Otto Loewi, this observation was not yet fully established for the mammalian heart. With the help of physostigmine to inhibit cholinesterases and atropine to prevent the untoward muscarinic effects of physostigmine, it was possible to ascertain, by biological tests, the appearance of acetylcholine in the coronary venous blood of the dog and cat during electrical stimulation of the peripheral end of the severed vagus nerves. To exclude extraneous influences, the heart-lung preparation of the dog was successfully used and yielded the same result (Feldberg and Krayer, 1933). In the intact circulation of the dog, reflex vagal effects caused by electrical stimulation of the carotid sinus nerve, or intravenous injection of epinephrine led to an increase in the concentration of acetylcholine in the coronary venous blood. Using an innervated heart-lung preparation with the head perfused from a donor dog, it was shown that the effect of epinephrine was due to blood pressure increase in the circulation of the perfused head and that the resulting physiological reflex vagal stimulation was capable of causing an increase in the concentration of acetylcholine in the coronary venous blood of the heart-lung preparation (Krayer and Verney, 1935).

## *Physostigmine and neostigmine*

The use of physostigmine to inhibit cholinesterases in the intact organism drew attention to the lack of quantitative information on the relationship between dose and intensity and duration of effect of this pharmacologically important substance. Inhibition of serum cholinesterase was chosen as an indicator for the quantitative determination of physostigmine in the blood in vivo. The time course of the inhibition was followed in detail after single intravenous doses in dogs. With continuous intravenous infusion a steady level of inhibited serum cholinesterase activity was reached within an hour and could be maintained for as long as the infusion lasted. Percentage rate of cholinesterase activity attained by a constant rate of infusion was reproducible and allowed quantitative definition of "eserinization" when employed for physiological experiments involving cholinergic mechanisms. The validity of determinations of inhibited enzymes was examined from the standpoint of the various methods which may be employed in such determinations. Combination of inhibitor with enzyme, destruction of inhibitor, dilution, displacement of inhibitor by substrate, and time were shown to be among the factors by which methods differ and which require proper correction (Krayer, Goldstein and Plachte, 1944). (These experiments were successful because they had initiated the fundamental studies of Straus and Goldstein (1943)[1] and Goldstein (1944)[2]).

The quantitative study was extended to Neostigmine USP ("Prostigmine"). The interactions of dose, route of administration, excretion, destruction, and plasma levels were investigated in dogs and also in patients suffering from myasthenia gravis The behav-

---

1  STRAUS, O. H. & GOLDSTEIN, A. (1943). Zone behavior of enzymes; illustrated by the effect of dissociation constant and dilution on the system cholinesterase-physostigmine. J. Gen. Physiol., 26, 559-585.

2  GOLDSTEIN, A. (1944). The mechanism of enzyme-inhibitor-substrate reactions; illustrated by the cholinesterase-physostigmine-acetylcholine system. J. Gen. Physiol., 27, 529-580.

ior of the cholinesterase-neostigmine-acetylcholine system was examined. As in the dog, also in patients predictable neostigmine levels can be achieved by continuous intravenous infusions at a constant rate. To depress plasma cholinesterase activity in equal small steps requires dose increments whose magnitude increases exponentially. This should also be true of tissue cholinesterases. The very wide range of doses required clinically can thus be explained (Goldstein, Krayer, Root, Acheson and Doherty, 1949).

## *Veratrum alkaloids*

Work on the veratrum alkaloids started with the reinvestigation of the cardiac action of veratrine, and confirmation, especially in the failing heart of the heart-lung preparation, of the digitalis-like action of this mixture of alkaloids (Krayer and Mendez, 1942). This prompted a search for pure substances, e.g,, veratridine, for further studies and led to a critical evaluation of the literature (Krayer and Acheson, 1946). Veratridine, a monoester of the tertiary alkamine veracevine, is one of the main alkaloids responsible for the effects of veratrine. Its action in the normal and failing heart (Moe and Krayer, 1943), its heart rate decreasing, predominantly vagal, effect in the innervated heart (Krayer, Wood and Montes, 1943), and its blood pressure decreasing, vasodilator action in the intact circulation (Moe, Bassett and Krayer, 1944) were analyzed. One of the important results of these studies was the clarification, by the use of a pure alkaloid, of the sites of action of the reflex decrease in heart rate and blood pressure which is characteristic of low doses of many of the tertiary alkamine esters of the veratrum alkaloids. In part, this reflex has its origin in sensory receptors of the heart itself (now called Bezold-Jarisch effect, see Krayer, 1961) and, in part, in other sensory areas of the aorta and its branches and in the pulmonary artery. Veratridine has become an important pharmacological tool in the search for, and investigation of, sensory receptors and in the study of the sodium channels of excitable biological membranes. Special attention was also given to protoveratrine (Krayer, Moe and Mendez, 1944) which consists of protoveratrine A and protoveratrine B, two chemically closely related tetraesters of the tertiary alkamine protoverine with very similar pharmacological properties. Because, on intravenous injection, the blood pressure decreasing action develops more slowly and lasts longer than that of veratridine, protoveratrine was introduced into the treatment of human hypertension (Meilman and Krayer, 1950, 1952; Krayer, 1958). Hypotensive veratrum alkaloids of polyester nature, such as the protoveratrines, continue to have therapeutic usefulness in acute hypertensive states (Krayer and Meilman, 1977).

The "veratrine response", a myotonic reaction of the amphibian and mammalian skeletal muscle, was given renewed attention using pure tertiary alkamine ester alkaloids, e.g., veratridine and various esters of the tertiary alkamine germine, for a systematic study of their veratrine-like (veratrinic) activity in the amphibian skeletal muscle. The study could be extended to the intact mammal because some substances, e.g., germine acetate, showed little or no hypotensive activity in doses which exhibited the characteristic veratrinic action on skeletal muscle. This suggested the use of such compounds for the treatment of myasthenia gravis (see Flacke et. al., 1966)[3].

The naturally occurring veratrum alkaloids belong to two different chemical groups, i.e., the tertiary alkamines and their esters, mentioned above, and the secondary alkamines. The first experiments with veratramine, a secondary alkamine of known structure, and which had never before been studied pharmacologically, led to the recognition of a novel group of substances possessing a heart rate decreasing activity entirely different from that of veratridine or other tertiary alkamine ester alkaloids (Krayer, 1949). It is a direct, selective action upon the pacemaker of the

---

3 FLACKE, W., CAVINESS, V. S. & SAMAHA, F. G. (1966). Treatment of myasthenia gravis with germine diacetate. New Engl. J. Med., 275, 1207-1214.

heart while the rate-decreasing effect of veratridine is predominantly of reflex vagal nature. This property of veratramine was named antiaccelerator activity because it is most striking if the heart rate is elevated above the normal level, and it is not prevented or abolished by atropine (Krayer, 1950). In the presence of veratramine, sympathomimetic amines exhibit full action upon the force of contraction, atrioventricular propagation time, functional and absolutely refractory periods of atrioventricular transmission, while their heart rate increasing action is reduced or abolished (Krayer, Mandoki and Mendez, 1951). This antiaccelerator property was also found in other secondary alkamines of the veratrum series (Krayer, 1950), and among the steroidal solanum alkaloids of secondary amine nature. It was obtained by partial synthesis from steroidal sapogenins and sex hormones by introduction of nitrogen into the molecule (Krayer, 1952). On the amphibian skeletal muscle, veratramine has very little, if any, veratrinic action; rather, like quinine, it is an antagonist to the veratrinic action of veratridine (Krayer and George, 1951).

## *Rauwolfia alkaloids*

The early investigations of the Rauwolfia alkaloid reserpine, used in the treatment of hypertension and as tranquilizing agent, were generally assumed to indicate that its various pharmacological effects were due to actions upon structures of the central nervous system. In 1955, the heart-lung preparation of the dog was used to challenge this assumption by exploring whether or not reserpine had direct actions upon the heart. There was a complex effect upon the rate of the heart beat. It was discovered that, in a relatively low dosage range, reserpine led to an increase in heart rate which developed gradually, reached a plateau and then slowly subsided. The effect was dose-dependent and resembled the action of epinephrine or norepinephrine infused continuously into the heart-lung preparation at a gradually increasing then decreasing rate (Krayer and Fuentes, 1956, 1958). The heart rate increase was due to intrinsic cardiac norepinephrine and was linked to norepinephrine depletion of the heart. Thus, it was absent in heart-lung preparations from dogs whose cardiac norepinephrine stores had been depleted prior to isolation of the heart (Krayer and Paasonen, 1957; Paasonen and Krayer, 1958; Waud, Kottegoda and Krayer, 1958). In the heart-lung preparation with normal norepinephrine stores, reserpine not only caused the chronotropic but also the the inotropic, dromotropic, and bathmotropic effects characteristic of the cardiac action of norepinephrine and other sympathomimetic amines. All these effects, which are mediated by norepinephrine, as well as the norepinephrine-depleting action, were found to be a property of the reserpine-type but not of the yohimbine-type Rauwolfia alkaloids (Innes, Krayer and Waud, 1958; Paasonen and Krayer, 1959).

After a dose of one milligram of reserpine had exerted its maximal heart rate increasing effect in the heart-lung preparation, no further increase could be obtained by the same or even a larger additional dose. On the contrary, the heart rate decreased and, by further cumulative doses, could be lowered in steps to the initial level, or below, in a manner which resembled the antiaccelerator action of veratramine (Krayer and Fuentes, 1958; Innes and Krayer, 1958).

# Selected bibliography


FELDBERG, W. & KRAYER, O. (1933). Das Auftreten eines azetylcholinähnlichen Stoffes im Herzvenenblut von Warmblütern bei Reizung der Nervi vagi. Arch. exp. Path. Pharmakol., 172, 170-193.

GOLDSTEIN, A., KRAYER, O., ROOT, M. A., ACHESON, G. H. & DOHERTY, M. A. (1949). Plasma neostigmine levels and cholinesterase inhibition in dogs and myasthenic patients. J. Pharmacol. exp. Ther., 96, 56-85.

INNES, I. R. & KRAYER, O. (1958). Studies on veratrum alkaloids. XXVII. The negative chronotropic action of veratramine and reserpine in the heart depleted of catecholamines. J. Pharmacol. exp. Ther., 124, 245-251.

INNES, I. R., KRAYER, O. & WAUD, D. R. (1958). The action of Rauwolfia alkaloids on the functional refractory period of atrioventricular transmission in the heart-lung preparation of the dog. J. Pharmacol. exp. Ther., 124, 324-332.

KRAYER, O. (1928). Über Verteilung und Ausscheidung des Jodes nach Zufuhr von Schilddrüsenstoffen. Arch. exp. Path. Pharmakol., 128, 116-125.

KRAYER, O. (1929). Die akute Kreislaufwirkung des Neosalvarsans. I. Mitteilung: Die Analyse der Kreislaufwirkung. Arch. exp. Path. Pharmakol., 146, 20-43.

KRAYER, O. (1930). Die akute Kreislaufwirkung des Neosalvarsans. II. Mitteilung: Über die Ursache der Kreislaufwirkung. Arch. exp. Path. Pharmakol., 153, 50-66.

KRAYER, O. (1931). Versuche am insuffizienten Herzen. Arch. exp. Path. Pharmakol., 162, 1-28.

KRAYER, O. (1949). Studies on veratrum alkaloids. VIII. Veratramine, an antagonist to the cardioaccelerator action of epinephrine. J. Pharmacol. exp. Ther., 96, 422-437.

KRAYER, O. (1950). Studies on veratrum alkaloids. XII. A quantitative comparison of the antiaccelerator cardiac action of veratramine, veratrosine, jervine and pseudojervine. J. Pharmacol. exp. Ther., 98, 427-436.

KRAYER, O. (1952). Antiaccelerator cardiac agents. J. Mount Sinai Hospital, 19, 53-69.

KRAYER, O. (1958). Veratrum alkaloids. In Pharmacology in Medicine, 2nd Ed. by V. A, Drill, Editor. Chapter 34, pp. 515-524. New York: McGraw-Hill.

KRAYER, O. (1961). The history of the Bezold-Jarisch effect. Arch. exp. Path. Pharmakol., 240, 361-368.

KRAYER, O. & ACHESON, G. H. (1946). The pharmacology of the veratrum alkaloids. Physiol. Rev., 26, 383-446.

KRAYER, O., GOLDSTEIN, A. & PLACHTE, F. L. (1944). Studies on physostigmine and related substances. I. Quantitative relation between dosage of physostigmine and inhibition of cholinesterase activity in the blood serum of dogs. J. Pharmacol. exp. Ther., 80, 8-30.

KRAYER, O. & FUENTES, J. (1956). Chronotropic cardiac action of reserpine. Federation Proceedings 15, 1462.

KRAYER, O. & FUENTES, J. (1958). Changes of heart rate caused by direct cardiac action of reserpine. J. Pharmacol. exp. Ther., 123, 145-152.

KRAYER, O. & GEORGE, H. W. (1951). Studies on veratrum alkaloids. XV. The quinine-like effect of veratramine upon the single twitch and upon the "veratrine response" of the sartorius muscle of the frog. J. Pharmacol. exp. Ther., 103, 249-258.

KRAYER, O., MANDOKI, J. J. & MENDEZ, C. (1951). Studies on veratrum alkaloids. XVI. The action of epinephrine and of veratramine on the functional refractory period of auriculo-ventricular transmission in the heart-lung preparation of the dog. J. Pharmacol. exp. Ther., 103, 412-419.

KRAYER, O. & MEILMAN, E. (1977). Veratrum alkaloids with antihypertensive activity. In Handbook of Experimental Pharmacology, Heffter-Heubner New Series., 39, Antihypertensive Agents. Editor F. Gross. Chapter 12, pp.547-570. Berlin, Heidelberg, New York· Springer-Verlag.

KRAYER, O. & MENDEZ, R. (1942). Studies on veratrum alkaloids. I. The action of veratrine upon the isolated mammalian heart. J. Pharmacol. exp. Ther., 74, 350-364.

KRAYER, O., MOE, G. K. & MENDEZ, R. (1944). Studies on veratrum alkaloids. VI. Protoveratrine: its comparative toxicity and its circulatory action. J. Pharmacol. exp. Ther., 82, 167-186.

KRAYER, O. & PAASONEN, M. K. (1957). Direct cardiac action of reserpine. Acta physiol. scand., 42, 88-89.

KRAYER, O. & RÜHL, A. (1931). Über die Wirkung einer reinen Gefäßerweiterung auf den Gesamtkreislauf. (Zur Wirkungsweise des Kallikreins). Arch. exp. Path. Pharmakol., 162, 70-85.

KRAYER, O. & SATO, G. (1928). Schilddrüsenwirkung und autonomes Nervensystem. Arch. Exp. Path. Pharmakol., 128, 67-81.

KRAYER, O. & VERNEY, E. B. (1935). Reflektorische Beeinflussung des Gehaltes an Azetylcholin im Blute der Coronarvenen. Arch. exp. Path. Pharmakol., 180, 75-92.

KRAYER, O., WOOD, E. H. & MONTES, G. (1943). Studies on veratrum alkaloids. IV. The sites of the heart rate-lowering action of veratridine. J. Pharmacol. exp. Ther., 79, 215-224.

MEILMAN, E. & KRAYER, O. (1950). Clinical studies on veratrum alkaloids. I. The action of protoveratrine and veratridine in hypertension. Circulation, 1, 204-213.

MEILMAN, E. & KRAYER, O. (1952). Clinical studies on veratrum alkaloids. II. The dose-response relations of protoveratrine in hypertension. Circulation, 6, 212-221.

MOE, G. K., BASSETT, O. L. & KRAYER, O. (1944) Studies on veratrum alkaloids. V. The effect of veratridine and cevine upon the circulation in anesthetized dogs with particular reference to femoral arterial flow. J. Phamacol. exp. Ther., 80, 272-284.

MOE, G. K. & KRAYER, O. (1943). Studies on veratrum alkaloids. II. The action of veratridine and cevine upon the isolated mammalian heart. J. Pharmacol. exp. Ther., 77, 220-228.

PAASONEN, M. K. & KRAYER, O. (1958) The release of norepinephrine from the mammalian heart by reserpine. J. Pharmacol. exp. Ther., 123, 163-160.

PAASONEN, M. K. & KRAYER, O. (1959). The content of noradrenaline and adrenaline in the rat heart after administration of Rauwolfia alkaloids. Experientia, XV/2, p.75.

WAUD, D. R., KOTTEGODA, S. R. & KRAYER, O. (1958). Threshold dose and time course of norepinephrine depletion in the mammalian heart by reserpine. J. Pharmacol. exp. Ther., 124, 340-346.

# *Books edited*

P. TRENDELENBURG (1934). Die Hormone. Ihre Physiologie und Pharmakologie. Volume 2. Edited by Otto Krayer. Berlin: Springer.

P. TRENDELENBURG's Grundlagen der allgemeinen und speziellen Arzneiverordnung.

(1931) Third edition by Otto Krayer. Berlin: F.C.W. Vogel.

(1938) Fourth edition by Otto Krayer. Berlin: F. C. W. Vogel.

(1952) Seventh edition by Otto Krayer and Manfred Kiese. Berlin, Göttingen, Heidelberg: Springer.

# Otto Krayer:
# Curriculum vitae

At the time of my birth, on October 22, 1899, my parents lived in the village of Köndringen im Breisgau in the today's federal state of Baden-Württemberg. My father, Hermann Krayer, was a farmer. My mother, Frieda, née Wolfsperger, was the daughter of an inn keeper.

Between the age of 6 and 10 I attended the primary school in Köndringen. Then followed six years of Realschule [i.e., a school oriented towards mathematics and science] in the neighbouring town Emmendingen and, in 1916, I entered the Oberrealschule in Freiburg i.Br. In 1917, before the end of the Obersekunda [the 11th school year] I was drafted into the army and served actively on the Western front from April to October 1918. At the beginning of 1919 I returned to the Oberrealschule in Freiburg i. Br. from which I graduated on July 19, 1919.

I began my medical studies in Freiburg. Then followed three semesters at the University of München, were I passed the preclinical examination. My clinical studies at the universities of Freiburg and Berlin were completed in 1924 with the Staatsexamen [final examination] in Freiburg i.Br. In 1925 the first half of my Medizinalpraktikantenjahr [year of internship] was devoted to experimental work under the supervision of the pharmacologist at Freiburg, Professor Paul Trendelenburg. The report of my work served as my dissertation. My obligatory six months of training in internal medicine were spent in the Medizinische Universitätsklinik of Freiburg, under the directorship of Professor Oscar De La Camp. I received my licence to practice medicine and my promotion to Dr.med. on January 1, 1926. Simultaneously I began my academic career as an Assistent [assistant] at the Department of Pharmacology of the University of Freiburg i.Br.

In October 1927 I followed Professor P. Trendelenburg to the Department of Pharmacology of the University of Berlin, was promoted to Oberassistent in 1928 and obtained my Habilitation [qualification as Lecturer in Pharmacology] in 1929. During Paul Trendelenburg's illness and after his death I was acting head of the Department of Pharmacology in Berlin from August 1, 1930, to the spring of 1932, i.e., until Professor Wolfgang Heubner took over the directorship of the department. In January 1932 I received the title of ausserplanmässiger ao. Professor.

At the beginning of 1933 I took leave of absence in order to complement my scientific training at the Department of Physiology of the University of Göttingen. A few weeks after my arrival in Göttingen this plan came to nothing, because of a dispute with the Prussian Kultusministerium[1] [Ministry of Education] concerning the chair of pharmacology in Düsseldorf which had become vacant after the dismissal of Professor Philipp Ellinger. Having been forbidden to enter any German university, I was forced to return to Berlin in order to be able to continue, with the help of private libraries, my literary work on the unfinished book by Paul Trendelenburg "Die Hormone II". The realisation that the changed political conditions made any academic future impossible, caused me to accept the offer of working space in the Department of Pharmacology of University College in London. A Rockefeller Fellowship enabled me to accept this offer. After

---

1 NISSEN, R. (1969). Helle Blätter-dunkle Blätter. Erinnerungen eines Chirurgen., 140-141. Stuttgart: Deutsche Verlagsanstalt. – REITER, M. & TRENDELENBURG, U. (1982). In memoriam Otto Krayer. Naunyn-Schmiedeberg's Arch. Pharmacol., 320, 1-2. – GOLDSTEIN, A. (1987). Otto Krayer 1899-1982. A Biographical Memoir.Biographical Memoirs, 57, 151-225. Washington, D. C.: The National Academy Press. – TRENDELEN-BURG, U. (1995). Otto Krayer und das "Gesetz zur Wiederherstellung des Berufsbeamtentums"(April 1933), DGPT Mitteilungen Nr.16, 33-34 Stuttgart: Wissenschaftliche Verlagsgesellschaft.

having finished the ongoing scientific work I left Germany on December 31, 1933 and began my work in the Department of Pharmacology, University College, London, in early January 1934.

In August 1934 I was offered the directorship of the Department of Pharmacology of the American University in Beirut. As Visiting Professor of Pharmacology I was head of this department during the academic years 1934/35, 1935/36 and 1936/37.[2]

In the autumn of 1937 I accepted an invitation by Harvard University, Cambridge, Massachusetts, U.S.A., and became Associate Professor of Pharmacology at Harvard Medical School, Boston, Massachusetts. Immediately after my arrival I applied for American citizenship. On July 27, 1939, I married in Boston Dr. med. Erna Ruth Philipp, a paediatrician emigrated from Germany. Our marriage remained childless.

At the beginning of the academic year 1939/40 I assumed the directorship of the Department of Pharmacology of Harvard Medical School, as the successor to emeritus professor Reid Hunt. I directed this department until September 1966, from 1939–51 as Associate Professor of Comparative Pharmacology, from 1951–54 as Professor of Pharmacology, from 1954–63 as Charles Wilder Professor of Pharmacology and from 1964–66 as Gustavus Adolphus Pfeiffer Professor of Pharmacology. I retired in September 1966.

After my retirement I assumed, for short periods, the following academic positions: Visiting Centennial Professor of Pharmacology, Howard University, Washington, D. C., in October, November and December 1966; Visiting Professor of Pharmacology, Stanford University, Palo Alto, California, in January,

---

2  FAWAZ, G. (1983). Cornerstones. A rare bird of passage alights on the AUB campus and stays on for three years. Otto Krayer (1899-1982) as I knew him. Medicus, 15, 10-15.

February and March 1968; Visiting Professor at the Department of Pharmacology and Toxicology of the Technical University of München, in May, June and July 1972; Visiting Professor of Pharmacology, University of Arizona, College of Medicine, Tucson, Arizona, since September 1972.

Tucson, Arizona, U.S.A.
November 21, 1972

Otto Krayer

# Acknowledgements

For his support during the work on Otto Krayer's manuscript I owe Ullrich Trendelenburg special thanks; all chapters profited from his critical comments.

Access to biographical sources was provided by Robert Domenjoz, Dieter Forst, Hans Haas, Joseph Hamacher, Arnold Hasselblatt, Karl Karzel, Heinz Lüllmann, as well as by Peter Heistracher, Otto Kraupp and Gabriele Schmidt in Wien.

With magnanimity Wolfgang Forth made available to me the treasures of the library and the archives of the Walther-Straub-Institute of the Ludwig-Maximilian-University in München.

Help, especially in my search for further literature, came from Hans-Josef Daleiden (Bayer AG), Wulf D. von Lucius, Wolfgang Wirth, and from the members of the Department of Pharmacology and Toxicology of the Technical University in München under the directorship of Franz Hofmann: Wolfgang Brandt, who found rather inaccessible texts, Wolfgang Vierling and Brigitte Dick, and especially Marianne Egetemeyer, who achieved the formal uniformity of the texts and put together the index.

The printing was supported by grants from Bayer AG and Bayer Vital GmbH, Germany.

To all of them sincere thanks are owed.

# List of Illustrations

Otto Krayer, in his 75th year, 1974 (Dept. of Pharmacology and Toxicology, Technical University, München)

Oswald Schmiedeberg and Rudolf Boehm (Archives of the Walther-Straub-Institute of the Ludwig-Maximilians-University, München)

Rudolf Boehm (München. med. Wschr., 1926, 73/II, 2170)

Arthur Heffter (Arch. exp. Path. Pharmakol., 1925, 105, I-V, 264-265)

Walther Straub, in his 60th year, 1934 (Dr. Peter Straub)

Oscar Gros, in his 64th year, 1941 (Deutsches Museum, München)

Joseph Schüller (Joseph Hamacher)

Fritz Külz (Cornelia Kroker)

Hermann Fühner, before his 60th year (Bayerische Staatsbibliothek)

Paul Trendelenburg, in his 33rd year, 1917 (Ullrich Trendelenburg)

August Wilhelm Forst, in his 65th year, 1955 (Dr. Dieter Forst)

Hellmut Weese (Bayer AG)

Conference of the Health Organisation of the League of Nations in Geneva 1925 (estate of Otto Krayer)

# Name Index

*This is one of three thousand and five hundred copies
printed on behalf of the National Committee
for distribution to participants at the IUPHAR Congress,
München, July 26–31, 1998*